Sidney Harris's background has afforded him an unusual position to write about diet and health. From his early years as a wholesaler and importer of fruit and vegetables in Covent Garden he passed through several other trades before becoming a bookshop owner in Hove, Sussex, in the early 1980's. It was in this guise that I first met him. Apart from the esoteric his bookshop stocked many popular titles and from this vantage point he could see the public's voracious appetite for diet books, and their search to have their unfounded beliefs reinforced.

The Royal College of Physicians recently published an important report: 'Nutrition and Patients - A Doctor's Responsibility.'

This report emphasis the importance of nutrition and in its own words is a "wake up call" to the medical profession.

From my own point of view as a clinician involved in nutrition for over twenty years and as a member of that same college, the need for a wake-up call for both doctors and the public alike has never been greater.

In that spirit, I commend this book to you. Read it and you should take away something for both your body and mind.

Dr Alan Stewart M.B..B.S. MRCP (U.K)

*"If you were to give every individual
the right amount of nourishment,
not too little, not too much, we will have found
the safest way to health."*
        - Hippocrates

Index

Page:

1	Part One Non-Food
2	Anti-Atkins
6	Core Cravings
7	The Evolutionary Diet
8	Zen
9	Staying Alive
10	Carbohydrates
20	People Power
25	Easily Influenced
26	Cause & Effect
28	Milk
30	Food Poisoning
31	Sugar
32	Caffeine
33	Salt
36	Food Intolerance
37	Dangerous Ingredients
38	Traditional Dangers
39	Microwaves
40	Non-Food
41	Shelf Life
42	Emotional Eating
45	Protein
48	The Bigger Picture
50	Pandemic Waiting to Happen
51	Spiritual Equation
52	Water
53	Part Two Real-Food
54	A Proven Diet
55	The Mediterranean Diet
56	Zen Two
57	Simple Changes
58	Human Proportions
59 to 97	The Nutrients In Real-Food
98	The Latter and The Former
99	The Price of Rice
100	The Same Old Story

Part One
Non-Food

"Sometime the voice of reason doesn't shout loudly enough!"
- Chinese Proverb

Anti-Atkins

In March 2000 the American Heart Association drafted an advisory paper warning the public about the dangers of high-protein diets. Explaining that, in the long term the saturated fat and cholesterol content of the diet will increase the risk of cardiovascular diseases, particularly heart attacks.

In August 2002 it was made clear to doctors that they faced possible legal action if they did not warn their patients about diets placing them at risk. The Atkins diet is a high animal protein diet combined with a very low carbohydrate intake. Fruit and vegetables contain carbohydrate, which initially completely excludes them from the Atkins diet, this is completely at odds with medical research of the last sixty years. The late Dr. Atkins admitted in a television program that there were no independent clinical trials to back up his theories; just amazing results from his own files.

Ten months after Dr. Atkins death in a report *mistakenly* released by New York's chief medical officer it was made public that Dr. Atkins the greatest exponent of his own diet was clinically obese and had a history of heart attacks, congestive heart failure and hypertension. This was reported on the front page of The Times on 11th February 2004.

When carbohydrates are removed from a diet, such as the Atkins diet, muscle mass is digested first, resulting in a quick weight loss in the early stages of the diet. The loss of this muscle mass sets up a chain reaction in the body. When muscle is broken down to liberate glucose to the brain it creates a dramatic water loss and an immediate weight loss. With the loss of muscle mass comes a loss of strength. In simple terms the diet sets up a form of self-cannibalisation.

Over forty per cent of the U.K population is made up of diabetics and people with kidney complaints. This section of the population should not contemplate the Atkins diet for one moment.

" You want my response to Atkins diet, saying his diet can lower your cholesterol and do all good things for your heart? You know what my response is? Bullshit!"

- Judith Stern
Professor of nutrition & internal medicine at Univ. of California.

Although Dr. Atkins first published his diet in the 1970's it lacked its main proponent - the amazing power of celebrity endorsement. A handful of nubile Hollywood starlets endorsed the diet on the strength of its fast initial weight loss - that amounted to them dropping one dress size, overshadowing the advice of the medical establishment.

In fairness to the late Dr. Atkins and his publishers they make it quite clear that anyone following the *suggestions* made in the Atkins diet should first seek medical advice, as they are not willing to take any responsibility for the long-term consequences.

For those who embarked on the Atkins diet without seeking medical advice, these are some of the known consequences which amount to a three-pronged attack on the body; firstly "gluco-neo-genesis" takes place, the making of glucose retrieved from glycogen stores within the muscles – including the heart muscle. In effect the body starts to consume lean body mass to create glucose. Essential potassium, magnesium and calcium are lost in urine and the autoimmune system is depressed placing a considerable strain on the kidneys, as a result of starving the body of carbohydrates.

The problem does not end there; the body now has to cope with the additional fat and protein advocated by the diet leading to long term problems from saturated fats, namely: heart disease, diabetes, colon cancer, prostate cancer, osteoporosis and hypertension. High intake of arachidonic acid found in beef, pork and dairy foods produce inflammatory chemicals that promote Crohn's disease, arthritis, gout and psoriasis.

This initial pincer attack on the body is followed by the third arm of the attack, the restriction of eating fruit, because of its carbohydrate content, means that the body is denied vital anti-oxidants that fight disease. This means that any potential medical problem will be exacerbated.

" Eating large amounts of high-fat foods for a sustained period raises the risk of coronary heart disease, diabetes, stroke and several types of cancer."
                                                    - American Heart Association.

3

In a report filed by Marian Burros in the New York Times, 18th January 2004, it stated that, Collette Heimowitz, a director of research and education for Atkins Nutritionals, is now telling health professionals that only 20 percent of dieter's calories should come from saturated fat. Atkins representatives said that Dr. Atkins always maintained that people should eat other food beside red meat, but had *"difficulty in getting the message out."* Collette Heimowitz, explained, *"... that's why we had to write another book, to get the story straight."*

Without being overly cynical, surely the original message could have been made succinct, years before millions of books had been sold.

Later in Marian Burros report she outlines the opinion of:

Dr. Frank M. Sacks at the Harvard Medical School of Public Health, *" What they are saying is ridiculous, the revision has nothing to do with science, it has to do with public relations and politics."*

It would now seem that Atkins Nutritionals, who reported $100 million in revenues in 2002, are fighting a rear guard action on their original standpoint of, *'eat as much saturated fat as you like,'* while mounting a full frontal attack on advocating a *'low carbohydrate diet.'*

If we take the current Atkins train of thought, to its logical conclusion, virtually all the food, high in carbohydrate, grown on earth is unnecessary, and the development of the human species over millions of years, was achieved on an ill conceived diet. It is difficult to separate the audacity from the arrogance!

In a study led by Dr. Judith Wurtmen at the Massachusetts Institute of Technology, it was found that eating starchy carbohydrates such as potatoes and bread, when part of a balanced diet, increased the brain's serotonin levels, maintaining equilibrium.

Dr.Wurtmen explained that some people were carbohydrate cravers and eating a lot of protein and fat as recommended on the Atkins diet could turn them into 'Emotional Zombies.'

Atkins Nutritionals, who have turned defending the indefensible into an art form, dispute the claim.

*" In my experience people on the Atkins diet are
prone to mood swings, anxiety and erratic behaviour."*
- Dr Cecilia Tregear
Specialist on effect of diet on hormone levels

What if you were to follow the obverse of the Atkins diet? Reduce meat and animal fat intake to a minimum and increase carbohydrate intake. What effect would this have on your body?

The effect of doing the exact opposite to the Atkins diet is quite enlightening, especially if you adhere to it for a prolonged period of time. You would lose weight and increase your life expectancy by seven years.

Of course, a claim of such magnitude has to be proven. Well the claim has been proven, beyond doubt - on a sample of forty eight million people over a period of fourteen years.

The fourteen-year period began in March 1940 and finished in June 1954. The guinea pigs in the experiment were the inhabitants of the United Kingdom. This was the period that rationing on meat and dairy foods existed due to World War Two. The amount of meat and dairy food that an Atkins dieter can eat in one day was not consumed in a month under the United Kingdom's rationing rules. Potato consumption rose by sixty-per cent. Indeed potatoes and root vegetables were the mainstay of the British diet. "Dig for Victory" was the motto of the day as the beleaguered inhabitants of the British Isles helped to grow their own vegetables. Children's diets were enhanced with cod liver oil. The results were well documented, a leaner and healthier population, whose life expectancy was increased by seven years.

In Strom and Jensen's, 'Mortality from Circulatory Diseases in Norway, 1940-45' the same effects were mirrored in a shorter period.

In 2003 as a direct consequence of the Atkins diet, potato consumption in Los Angeles, the heartland of Atkins dieters, fell by sixty per cent. Of course this is an extreme statistic in a place where fad diets traditionally elicit an over exaggerated reaction.

Potato consumption in the United Kingdom is falling four per cent, year on year. Bankruptcies amongst potato growers are increasing and the long-term effect could be devastating to our food chain, if the potato, one of the staple foods of the western world, is decimated by people following a diet based on pseudo science.

"Disciples of the Atkins diet are gambling with their future health."
  - Dr. Susan Jebb   Medical Research Council Cambridge

Core Cravings

The most misguided of all theories is that the lack of willpower is the reason people become overweight. The potent factor that defeats an overweight person's attempts at dieting is the primal need to survive.

Anyone who sets out on a diet that does not sate the core cravings developed through evolution is attempting the impossible. Our basic craving is for Fat, Sugar and Salt regardless of how they are disguised.

Our core cravings are part of our very being, any attempt at ignoring these cravings results in an inner struggle that causes anguish and stress compensated by overeating. The only diet to which we are suited is the diet that created us; the diet that made us into the human beings we are today. Where so called *revolutionary* diets fail; the evolutionary diet has worked since the dawn of man. We exist because all the food we ever needed in order to exist was in close proximity to us. Our development was paralleled by the food around us, it was a predetermined and homogeneous process.

Alchemy is as useless in the production of food as it was in the production of gold; we cannot improve on natural raw material, only deplete it.

The cult of non-food has taken hold. Manufactured and processed *foods* overwhelm us at every turn in the supermarket. Putrescent meat products and dairy foods have developed a mythological status as being natural and healthy food for human beings.

The benefits of eating real-food as opposed to non-food have evaded us. Addiction to non-foods has become commonplace and food obsession has become part of our culture.

All we need to do to reach and maintain our optimum weight is to exercise moderately and enjoy real-food in human proportions.

To devise a diet for you, your unique needs have to be understood completely, and the only person who can truly understand your needs is you. You have to be the architect of your own existence.

There is a complete industry promoting fads and fashions in food, once you regain control of the situation you can ignore them.

" If you don't control your own mind, someone else will."
- John Allston

The Evolutionary Diet

In the last 50 years achieving the optimum diet has been something of a Holy Grail. New fad diets appear daily in the tabloids; diet books appear weekly, including non-diets claiming that diets do not work, while imparting yet another diet. If you were to read at random - twenty diet books from the thousands produced you would be confused and no wiser about what, in effect, should be simplicity itself; how a human being can gain nourishment, reach and maintain their optimum weight, without a struggle or harmful side effects.

There are diets available at the moment based on your astrological sign, your blood group and the shape of your head. You might decide that an amalgamation of these three might seem feasible and create yourself a fourth diet. Re-vamping old diets is quite a common practice – diets such as, high fibre, low fat, low carbohydrate, food combining, once a week detox, banana and milk, cabbage soup or that old stager; counting calories until you develop a compulsive behaviour disorder; all of these diets are recycled every few years. The new danger is counting carbohydrates until an eating disorder develops.

It is no wonder that dieters become demoralised by an overload of conflicting information that invariably has little to do with reality.

It takes no genius to draw together all of the best aspects of diet that human beings have thrived upon for thousands of years. We just need to look objectively at the diverse eating habits of the world's population, past and present, and what is a wholesome and healthy diet becomes obvious.

In the United States in 2003, dieters spent more than a billion dollars on quick fix diets, meal replacement drinks and potions that are reputed to be appetite suppressants. If they achieved any success at all, it was invariably short lived as ninety-per cent of all dieters regain their weight loss. You can be sure that the majority, of the ten percent, who maintained their weight loss, followed a sensible eating plan based on nutrition not the lack of it.

" Unfortunately there are too many advertisements
for scientifically impossible weight loss products. "
  - T. J. Muris   U.S. Federal Trade Commission

Zen

Over two thousand years ago Zen Buddhist monks developed a simple diet that consisted of eating only food grown in close proximity to where they lived. Anyone cured of hay fever by eating local grown honey will have some understanding of their rationale.

At the turn of the twentieth century George Ohsawa became ill with tuberculosis, which was at that time an incurable disease. As so many people do when they become ill, Ohsawa looked to diet to cure him; turning to the diet of the Zen Buddhist monks, he was successful in finding a cure.

Ohsawa introduced this diet, the diet of the Zen Buddhist monks, to the west; it became known as the Macrobiotic Diet.

We are light years away from these ancient Zen Buddhist monks who achieved a balance of yin and yang, the negative and positive forces, through meditation and diet. We have lost all semblance of simplicity by allowing ourselves to be swept along by any change the food manufacturers and supermarkets decide is more profitable for them. We are easily coerced into buying non-food.

There is far more depth to a Macrobiotic Diet than just ensuring that food does not go on unnecessary journeys; there is a resounding spiritual depth to it. Whereas we in the west are hardly in tune with the universe and our environment, exponents of a true Macrobiotic Diet, become attuned to the natural order of existence. The Macrobiotic Diet closely parallels that of fish eating vegans, a pesco vegan diet.

It is no easy task attempting to apply eastern philosophy and diet to the west, but there are valuable lessons to be learnt from a culture that has thrived on the same diet for over two thousand years, enjoying both physical and mental health. Especially when you compare it to the diet we have adopted over the last fifty years that has brought us obesity and illness.

We are in the fortunate position to be able to develop an eclectic diet that is fundamental to our needs, based on the diets of population's that have thrived.

" Enlightenment doesn't care how you get there." - Thaddeus Golas.

Staying Alive

If you were to embark on a fat free diet, no matter how promising it might seem - your brain, which incidentally is made up of seventy-five per cent fat, has an agenda of its own. It will not take part in your attempt to undermine your own system.

The first priority of your autonomic system is to keep you alive. Your body needs fat to regenerate your cells. The chemistry of the body is not predisposed to reconvert fat originally stored for energy to regenerate the body's cells. Twenty five per cent of the food eaten in a normal diet goes into the production of brain cells. Furthermore, your sense of sight and smell alert your autonomic system, of which you have no conscious control, to the fact that there is food all around you. Trying to impose the idea of starvation on your survival system is unacceptable. It's too much like suicide. The body will have none of it and redoubles your craving. Your willpower is just an idea but your craving is real. This is where your *willpower* is short-circuited.

If in the past you have blamed yourself for lack of willpower, because of failed attempts at dieting, you owe yourself an apology. But do not apologise too quickly if you are not taking at least twenty to thirty minutes exercise every day. Exercise is an area where your willpower can make all the difference. For those who are not exercising regularly; ease into it, walk a little, swim a little and take up yoga. The gentle stretching exercises of yoga are ideal for all ages; a few weeks of yoga can bring about a marked increase in fitness. A few months of yoga will wipe out years of inactivity.

Exercise is an essential part of the equation. Regular exercise raises your metabolism so that you burn fuel (calories) even when you are resting. Exercise increases your blood flow, strengthening your heart its blood vessels and your bones. This increased blood flow insures that the myriad of running repairs your body undergoes, twenty-four hours a day, can be performed at optimum level. Rigor mortis is not for the living.

" To get back my youth I would do anything in the world except exercise, get up early, or be respectable." - Oscar Wilde

Carbohydrates

The World Health Organisation recommends that we eat a diet rich in carbohydrates. Carbohydrates are essential to our existence, they not only power our bodies they also contain valuable minerals, (electrolytes) such as calcium, magnesium, potassium and sodium that carry messages from our brain to our muscles at the speed of thought.

The speed of thought varies from one person to another, we expect people in their twenties to react faster than people in their fifties.

The way to slow the reactions of a twenty-year old, down to those of a fifty-year old, is to lower their carbohydrate intake.

Indeed, not only will you slow down their reaction time and deplete their stamina, you will also induce cramp in their muscles that are starved of calcium, potassium, magnesium and sodium. Effectively without carbohydrates, you not only slow down but you seize up.

Anyone who has spent a day in an Olympic village will tell you that, Olympic athletes, regardless of the fact that many of them are meat eaters, also eat lots of fruit, vegetables, bread, pasta, grains and pulses. They load up with carbohydrates, aware that they cannot function without fuel.

There have of course been many vegetarian and vegan Olympic champions in all disciplines; 6 times gold medal winner Carl Lewis is a vegan. At the highest level in all fields of sport, vegetarian and vegan athletes excel. From Paavo Nurmi, long distance runner, 9 Olympic golds and 12 world records to Keith Holmes world middleweight-boxing champion and Peter Hussing European super heavyweight-boxing champion; just to mention a few. All of these athletes compound the proof that carbohydrates are essential, and dispel the myth that meat is a necessary *food* to build muscle - and for sheer endurance, look to Sixto Linares, 24-hour triathlon world record holder.

There are of course countless other non-meat eating athletes who excel, including Martina Navratilova, 9 times Wimbledon tennis champion, whose reflexes and stamina, as she approaches her fifties, leave most twenty-year olds in the shade.

You might feel that you need meat to get you through the cold winter months, Nicky Cole the first woman to reach the North Pole managed to reach her frozen destination on a vegetarian diet.

Fifteen years ago the incidence of coronary heart disease in Finland was the worst in Europe, as only three in ten Finns took any regular exercise. Appalled by the situation the Finnish government took concerted action to make their small population of five million understand the fatal danger of a sedentary lifestyle. The Finns heeded the warning and forty per cent, two million, hitherto sedentary people, took up regular exercise, resulting in a dramatic fall in the incidence of coronary heart disease. These figures are all the more encouraging when you take into account that the average age of Finns has markedly increased in the last fifteen years. Age is no barrier to taking moderate exercise.

In a 2003 survey the European Commission found that 12 percent of Britons said that they would struggle to walk five hundred yards. Whereas only 4.2 percent of Finns said they would struggle to go the same distance. Finland achieved the best score in Europe - Great Britain's score was the worst.

In essence, to start exercising, you do not need membership to an expensive gym or the services of a personal trainer, as used by Hollywood starlets who endorse fad diets.

In losing weight, time must not be your enemy. You have to realise that it takes three months of sensible eating and moderate exercise to lose approximately a stone in weight.

Once you realise this fundamental truth about safe weight loss, you have no unrealistic expectations and the whole process becomes much easier and you can relax, as time is on your side, there is no impossible deadline to achieve.

If you lose one to one and a half pounds in weight, per week, while eating a diet that makes you healthier and stronger, you are on the right track. If your diet satisfies you so much that you do not have cravings for the wrong foods; the profound side effect is that you develop a predilection for healthy eating; hopefully for life.

If there were a short cut to losing weight, the epidemic of obesity, which has struck the western world, would not have taken such control.

" It's not that some people have willpower and some don't
it's that some people are ready to change. "
    -   Dr. James Gordon M.D

A holistic change has to take place. Nobody can survive for any amount of time on what they perceive to be a diet. The notion is alien to us because we associate the word diet with denying ourselves the food we crave. To most of us a diet is something of a penance for having put on the weight in the first place. There is a lot of baggage attached to the word 'diet'. Of course there is the fantasy diet that sheds fourteen pounds in as many days, so that you can show up at that party in a fortnight looking svelte and fit. These misguided notions are universal to the overweight.

Apart from the psychological aftermath of failing to adhere, for any amount of time, to a fad diet and the damage caused by the poor nutritional values of these diets; there is the disastrous yo-yo effect on your metabolism created by on and off dieting. Your metabolism is geared for your survival, as with every other aspect of your body.

Your metabolism is a primal mechanism; it takes the famine-feast cycle at its face value. Not self-inflicted, but something inflicted upon you by the environment.

Continuous on-and-off dieting turns you into a fat storing entity. Your metabolism insures that the next time feast is followed by famine your body will have extra reserves of fat to survive. Any diet that cannot be adhered to for life is potentially dangerous as it misinforms your metabolism that food supplies in the outside world are sporadic. Subsequently fat reserves are optimised to ensure your survival; you become a slow burner of fuel. Crash diets reduce your calorie burning capacity by up to thirty per cent.

Apart from erratic eating patterns having a detrimental effect on your metabolism, erratic exercise patterns have a similar effect.

Infrequent bouts of sustained exercise that are not part of a regular routine fool your metabolism into conserving fat stores so that you have a ready supply of energy whenever you need it.

Indeed, the best recipe for slowing down your metabolism would be to go on a fad diet that you cannot sustain, have a game of squash once a fortnight and take up drinking alcohol; as your body's metabolism drops by up to seventy per cent after drinking alcohol.

" Everything is connected, no one thing can change by itself! "
- Paul Hawken

What is the antidote? How do you bring your body's metabolism back to equilibrium? It's simple, become consistent! Firstly try to get eight hours sleep each night. Less than five hours sleep a night induces the body to over-produce insulin and promote fat storage.

Ensure that you eat breakfast - it is the most important meal of the day, speeding up your metabolism that slowed down as you slept.

Eat little and often. After four hours without food your energy efficient body starts to conserve energy. By eating every four hours you re-crank your metabolism because food digestion and its absorption starts the energy burning process. You also have the advantage of small meals being easier to digest.

Exercise regularly, twenty to thirty minutes each day, brisk walking, swimming and gentle stretching exercises. There is also an excellent side effect to exercise; many weight problems are the result of underlying depression – regular light exercise helps to lift mild to moderate depression in just a few weeks.

Just as it took time and many failed diets to fool your metabolism into unnecessary fat storage. It will take time to reset your body's thermostat. A diet has to be sustainable for life otherwise it is just a stepping-stone to a further weight increase. There is no short cut. Complete equilibrium is the answer.

Every time you attempt the impossible you diminish your resolve. I'm sure that you have never achieved anything in life that was not directly related to common sense. If you have a realistic goal you will achieve it! Given the choice each of us would choose as an optimum diet, a diet that nourishes us to the maximum without us having to bother too much about its preparation, as simple a diet as possible - an enjoyable way of eating for life.

The concept of eating in human proportions will eventually override any calorie counting obsessions that you may have developed in the past. The diets you failed at were not your fault. They were faulty diets based on the assumption that you could exist on non-foods.

The easiest way to eradicate negative obsessions is to replace them with positive obsessions that enhance your wellbeing.

" Metabolism is somewhere in your body,
but nobody knows exactly where!" - Jackie Mason.

Our agenda is simple. We want to eat only the best food available, containing every nutrient, vitamin and mineral we need, while ensuring that we do not have a craving for fat, sugar and salt the villains of the piece. In the words of the song - we are trying to *"accentuate the positive and eliminate the negative."*

Before we eliminate the villains let us take a closer look at them. First we take a look at fat – the fat you find in meat, saturated fat, the fat that takes the blame for high cholesterol, heart attacks, cancer and numerous other diseases.

Animals in the wild have a very different physiology to us. The hydrochloric acid in the stomachs of carnivores, needed to digest meat, is twenty times stronger than that of human beings. Carnivores can easily digest meat, as their intestinal tract is a quarter of the length of that of a human being. Carnivores will eat virtually anything that moves, their life is ostensibly simple; they lurk at the waterhole and hope that eventually some fresh food in the form of meat will turn up. The meat these animals eat has a lot going for it. It's fresh unadulterated by hormones and antibiotics and, of course, it is lean, not having spent its life being force fed with anything that would ensure a fast weight gain; provided you are a carnivore, this meat is excellent. Seeing one animal tear another to pieces is repellent to most of us. The omnivore of today does not equate the steak in the supermarket with the slaughtering of an animal. The steak in the supermarket satisfies a developed craving, not a need; its hidden toxic content is out of sight and mind.

Man turned to eating meat in the last Ice Age for survival. Dire necessity turned man into an omnivore; he had no choice. Palaeolithic man's penchant for meat is over exaggerated; archaeologists have determined the Palaeolithic diet consisted of less than 20% meat.

Throughout the ages our ancestors faced famine many times whereas, we in the western world, are now faced with abundance.

Our survival depends on us returning to the food that was instrumental in our evolution, the food that initially nourished us, the food our bodies were specifically designed for.

> *" Feeding on the carcass of a slain animal*
> *has something of a bad taste about it.*   -   Leo Tolstoy

While there are still those who would disagree with Darwin, we are descendants of the great apes. Orang-utans and humans shared a common ancestor. Our DNA is only two percent different to the great apes whereas our DNA differs greatly from any other living omnivores or carnivores.

Unlike carnivores the great apes do not gorge themselves, they are highly selective in what they eat. They eat little and often, they chew their food and enjoy it, apart from fruit they eat seeds, nuts and selected roots. There is no doubt that our digestive systems are far closer to those of the great apes than carnivores. One definitive characteristic we have in common with apes is that they are the only other species that can see in colour, an essential asset in the search for fruit and berries. Like primates we need a regular source of vitamin C, whereas carnivores produce vitamin C internally.

Eating meat does not correlate with longevity; lions and tigers live for only ten years. One thing true carnivores have in common is that they sweat through their tongues - humans do not! The saliva of humans and the higher species of apes is alkaline – whereas the saliva of carnivores is acidic.

Our initial perception tends to leave us thinking that we have evolved rather than that we are still evolving. In the millions of years that it has taken us to evolve we have gone down many dead-ends. We either solved potential problems at the time or were decimated as a consequence. Our ancestors, having learnt valuable lessons, ensured our survival. Evolution is a slow and ongoing process, we are still travelling, we definitely haven't arrived.

To evolve into the *astute* characters we are today we were driven by our intuitive need to survive. Unfortunately the basic instinct that brought us this far is fast becoming alien to us. We no longer search for food. In actuality we do not really buy our food; we have it sold to us. We are victims of sales campaigns; this turn of events could easily be our next evolutionary dead-end. We are at the mercy of food manufacturers and their advertising. Regaining control is our best option for survival

"We will now discuss in a little more detail
the struggle for existence." - Charles Darwin

Whereas our distant ancestors in critical times needed to become carnivores to survive, we do not! Indeed, when our ancestors became carnivores the meat they ate was very different to the adulterated meat sold today, it contained CLA, conjugated linoleic acid an anti-carcinogenic that actively plays a part in weight control. The fitness developed by the strenuous activity of hunting also has to be taken into account. Unless you take up hunting in the wild, you are not going to find the kind of meat you *think* you need. In addition when meat is cooked it produces heterocyclic amines, cancer causing chemicals.

The blatant truth is, apart from added antibiotics, hormones, steroids, tenderisers and whatever else might have found its way into the meat, it also happens to be filled with saturated fat one of the biggest killers in the western world. Saturated fat is solid at room temperature whereas unsaturated fat is liquid.

The living counterparts of our Ice Age ancestors; live today in the harshest conditions on earth, in the arctic area of the Russian Federation, which stretches nearly half way around the world. They herd reindeer, which is their prime source of food. Reindeer meat is extremely low in saturated fat, 3.5 percent and contains more CLA than meat reared for *food* in the west. Lean beef in the west is 9.5 percent saturated fat. (Source of percentages Swanson 1990)

In as much as 'humans are what they eat' so are animals. Reindeer feed mainly on reindeer moss that grows just beneath the snow; this moss is actually a lichen half alga, half fungi, abundant in carbohydrates and vitamins. By courtesy of evolution, reindeer live on a custom made diet, far different to the synthetic concoctions fed to animals in the west, specifically designed to increase their weight.

Reindeer are killed and stored in freezing conditions, so putrefaction is not an issue, much as it wasn't when our distant ancestors started eating meat in the Ice Age.

The reindeer herders, due to the harshness of their existence and the restricted nutrients in their diet, notwithstanding, the meat they eat is less dangerous than meat reared in the west, had until twenty years ago a life expectancy of only fifty-five-years. Their already short life expectancy has been further reduced by ten-years, as they have no immunity to the respiratory diseases, brought to them by the recent influx of outsiders - drawn by the rich mineral deposits in the area.

The studies implicating meat in heart disease and cancer grow as fast as the mortality rate from these diseases. In general many people seem to think that these diseases happen to other people and they personally have some kind of immunity. Much the same as people disregard the warning on cigarettes which implicitly states that 'smoking kills.' Unfortunately there are no warnings on meat!

Although there are vast lobbies for the promotion of dairy foods, manufactured foods and meat, you will rarely see the vegan or vegetarian point of view expounded with any voracity.

The vast majority of doctors tell their patients to cut down on meat, as they are quite aware that invoking change is difficult, people become very fixed in their ways, especially where food is concerned.

Transition is not easy, but when the reason for transition is to improve your health and that of your family, it has to be considered deeply, the ultimate approach is to welcome transition.

In a study by Harvard scientists they found that women who ate beef, lamb or pork as their main meal daily, had two and a half times more risk of developing colon cancer than those who ate meat less than once a month.

We need fat in our diet otherwise we cannot function, but the fat we need has to have a positive effect. Animal fats cannot be contemplated, as they are dangerous.

To understand the dangers of saturated fat we must have a basic understanding of cholesterol - of which there are two types:

The very good is HDL cholesterol, High Density Lipoproteins, the liver produces this HDL cholesterol, essential to make hormones in our bodies and create cells.

The very bad is LDL cholesterol, Low Density Lipoproteins. The liver also produces this from saturated fat found in: meat, the skin of poultry, dairy products, palm oil, eggs, sausages, pies and manufactured food containing saturated fat.

" It is my view that the vegetarian manner of living
by its purely physical effect on the human temperament
would most beneficially influence the lot of mankind."
-   Albert Einstein

The ill effects of LDL cholesterol are manifold but the biggest risk is heart disease. The cholesterol in question, a waxy substance, clogs and narrows the arteries. Some people are more prone to cholesterol genetically; lack of exercise also plays its part. Smoking and stress also raise cholesterol levels. High LDL cholesterol levels must be reduced.

Would food producers have us believe that they are ignorant of the fact that thousands of tons of saturated fat are being pumped into the food chain? It has the effect of a lethal poison, but there is no law against it and no government warning on the food relating to its dangers. People unwittingly feed it to their children believing they are giving them nourishing food.

This is far from new information, it has been known for years. The American Heart Association made this information available over forty years ago.

Hopefully the U.K government will soon bring in legislation that makes food producers and manufacturers indicate the exact amount of saturated fat content. But in essence, the true answer to the problem is to avoid saturated fat completely.

There should be a hefty tax on potentially dangerous foods, much as there is on tobacco. This could go directly to funding hospitals where many of the people who eat this food unfortunately end up. This tax, by its very nature, would reward people who eat a healthy diet.

Olive oil protects the arteries and lowers the bad LDL cholesterol without lowering the good HDL cholesterol. It reduces blood pressure and is instrumental in regulating blood sugar it is also a potent antioxidant containing vitamin A and E, helping the body fight disease.

Olive trees live for thousands of years. In one olive grove in Greece fossilised leaves have been found that date back 40,000 years. Indeed, the olive tree that grew in Plato's back yard, over two thousand years ago is still alive. Plato was a vegetarian, as were: Ovid, Aristotle, Socrates and the father of modern medicine Hippocrates.

" As to diseases make a habit of two things –
to help, or at least to do no harm. "
                                                - Hippocrates

We truly are what we eat, drink and inhale. Those who overindulge and eat the wrong food, look and feel jaded. They punish themselves at a cellular level. Faulty thinking prevails and potential health problems are ignored. There is a large proportion of society that appears to be devoted to its own destruction. Almost every obese person you speak to has intentions of doing something about their condition on that amazing tomorrow that never arrives. Indeed, the obese pay into pensions funds at the same rates as the lithe and fit, they aspire to a healthy retirement, but the sad truth is that the obese are far less likely to collect than their fitter counterparts. Why would a person knowingly shortening their lifespan bother to pay into a pension fund?

There are few people that do not know the effects of scurvy, the disease caused by insufficient vitamin C.

Disease of the gums and teeth and bleeding into mucous membranes are symptoms that occur within a couple of months. One of the lesser-known later effects is that healed wounds and lesions, that are years old, reopen. This disease and many others are fostered by pursuing the obverse of nourishing the body with the vital nutrients it needs.

Therefore vitamin C and every other vitamin and nutrient are paramount to your wellbeing. Just knowing these facts is not enough you actually have to do something about it!

In three months time you will have changed. Every cell in your body will have replicated itself; each cell will have copied itself *almost* perfectly, and *almost* is the operative word for, had each cell been able to copy itself exactly you would not age. To draw an analogy, if you were to make photocopies of this page from each ongoing photocopy eventually, over a period of time, you would have only a faded likeness of the original. Although we cannot stop ageing; by eating the right nutrients, we can postpone ageing, in much the same way as the overweight postpone doing anything about their life-threatening situation. The body's ability to repair itself with the help of good nutrition is truly amazing.

" Almost all aspects of life are engineered at the molecular level and without understanding molecules we can only have a very sketchy understanding of life itself." - Francis Crick.

People Power

On the 25th February 2004, Nick Stace, campaign director for the Consumers' Association said the following in a press release:

"Obesity and diet-related diseases are now seen as Britain's biggest killer. But in response to this government and the food industry have produced consultations and consultations about consultations.

They have produced half-baked and half-hearted initiatives and ideas that all add up to nothing."

The Consumers' Association, which has seven hundred and fifty thousand members, is demanding that the Government set up a nutrition council. They are also asking for a ban to be enforced on all foods high in fat, sugar and salt in an effort to reduce obesity, which reduces life expectancy by an average of nine years.

If children were given one week of intensive, nutritional education, every year, we could guarantee them a healthier life and save the National Health Service billions of pounds in the future.

Children are brainwashed by junk food advertising on television, and there is absolutely no counterbalance. Supermarkets place colourful packets of nutritionally-bankrupt, breakfast foods on the lower shelves; using the cynical expedient of popular cartoon characters to entice children who can barely walk.

Manufacturers of non-foods have become so complacent with the fact that anything they package will be accepted that they keep pushing the boundaries. The more consumers prove themselves gullible the greater the price they are being made to pay in every respect.

Hopefully the consumer's acceptance will turn to anger, when they eventually decide that they can no longer tolerate their children's health being jeopardised.

It really is time for each and every one of us to put a stop to the lunacy by refusing to buy non-food. We only want unrefined real-food that is unadulterated. If we leave non-food on the shelves we will not have to wait for government legislation to stop the madness.

" Change often makes accepted customs into crimes."
Mason Cooley.

According to U.K. official figures one in five adults and thirteen percent of teenagers are clinically obese. The Government, who state they are finding it difficult to educate the public on food, estimate that in ten years time a quarter of the population will be obese. Independent reports make the projected figures far worse. Obesity has surpassed epidemic levels and continues to rise.

History will look upon us as a generation that lost its way in the supermarket. A people so easily led that they would buy anything the food manufacturers wanted to sell them. A population willing to pay many times the true price for food depleted of its original nutrients; a society regarded by its government as too dense to be educated in the preparation of a nourishing meal.

The figure of twenty percent of the population being obese was relatively easy for the government to ascertain. Of this ten million or so obese people it is much harder to determine how many are overweight due to eating the wrong food and how many due to emotional eating; and how many are suffering from both problems. In fact most obese people would like to find out into which category they actually fall.

If the government feel they have not the wherewithal to educate the public about food, how far out of their depth would they be if they contemplated tackling any underlying psychological problems that exist in part of the population. Negative mood is attributed to the main psychological reason for overeating; probably why the government prefers to blame overeating on poor education, than contemplate that a tract of the population may have underlying psychological problems.

One of the basic problems is that we are regarded first and foremost as consumers, hostage to the ongoing development of the food industry. There is no great conspiracy; this is just the unfortunate way things have been allowed to develop.

The problem the food industry now faces is that many of their products are shortening consumer's lives. In the long term, losing regular paying customers is not cost effective.

Consumer power is awesome - we can actually change the world by changing our diet. What other option do we have?

" The absence of alternatives clears the mind marvellously."
- Henry Kissinger

"We are at an absolutely fascinating moment in human evolution."
Was the opinion of Professor Andrew Prentice when he addressed the British Association for the Advancement of Sciences at their annual meeting at Leicester University 2003, where he elucidated on child couch potatoes:

" We have figured out ways of farming our fields without having to put in human labour, the same in factories where everything is done for us by robots, in the home we have gadgets to do almost everything.

Link that up with the seduction of TV viewing and Internet use and you have an explosive package. It's going to have massive consequences on our health and a massive effect on our health budget. Will parents outlive their children? Yes! When the offspring become grossly obese." Professor Prentice went on to say, *" Angina and heart attacks are going to be occurring in these children in the future. It is alarming that type two diabetes once described as adult onset diabetes, was now being reported by paediatric clinics."*

There could be no greater portent of evolution going down a dead end than children dying before their parents.

Professor Prentice concluded by telling the conference:
" Fast food and sedentary lifestyles are to blame. It's fifty-fifty, fast foods are likely to be implicated because they contain a lot of fat. The response to the high-energy, aggressively marketed foods and the sedentariness induced by TV is a pandemic of obesity. Even if a miracle drug was discovered to treat the problem, the cost of treating the sixty per-cent of the population who are overweight would be unimaginably huge." In conclusion Professor Prentice said: *"We are at an absolutely fascinating moment in human evolution. It's parallel with the increase in height two centuries ago as we pulled out of the desperate diet of the Middle Ages. Now we are going outwards in terms of girth, rather than increasing height. The important difference is that while the increase in height was beneficial the reverse is true of obesity."*

Anyone who has broken a limb and had to endure the months of being incapacitated in a plaster cast understands, all too well, the meaning of atrophy. When a muscle is not used - it dies. The integrity of our physiology relies on regular exercise.

" To wish to be well is part of becoming well. " - Seneca

Recently the U.S. Surgeon General David Satcher outlined the figures: *"Three Hundred Thousand Americans a year are dying from weight related illnesses."* It does not take much thought to realise that if the death toll is so high, the amount of people suffering chronically from weight related illnesses is a human catastrophe. After giving out these figures the Surgeon General went on to say: *"How to solve this problem is vexing, as warnings from health officials go unheeded."* World experts are in agreement, to quote the U.S. Surgeon General yet again: *" People eat more calories than they work off, shunning fruit and vegetables for super sized junk foods."*

The greatest false economy is super sized junk food. In diners and restaurants in the United States, in the last thirty years, portion sizes have doubled and tripled, as a sales gimmick to persuade people that they are getting *value*. Subsequently the average person has lost any conception of what a human portion of food should be. The official figures show that hundreds of thousands of people are dying because they have no idea of when to stop eating, having been coerced into overeating by cynical sales gimmicks.

In the United Kingdom the junk food market is worth fifteen billion pounds a year. The originators of junk food - the United States, can *boast* a junk food market worth over one hundred and twenty five billion dollars a year.

Feeding the population of the western world on junk food and then filling them with drugs to counteract heart disease, diabetes and the myriad of other diseases brought on by obesity only benefits the big food manufacturers and drug companies.

The problem is getting worse and independent medical experts believe that if the current trend prevails seventy five per cent of the U.K. population will be obese in fifteen years; a figure far higher than the government's already abysmal prediction. Tomorrow does not look too rosy, especially for those who continue to put off modifying their diet for sometime-never.

" A single death is a tragedy,
a million deaths are a statistic. "
- Joseph Stalin.

It can easily be argued that some of the amazing advances medical science has made in the last fifty years would not have occurred had it not had to fight the pandemic of diseases that obesity causes. This might well be true, but what an absurd life to lead, knowingly eating food that will one day lead to a heart transplant. With the donor of the organ, quite likely to be the same species of animal whose saturated fat caused the initial problem.

Most of us know that clearing rain forests causes global warming. At this very moment rain forests are being cleared and grass planted to feed vast herds of cattle, reared to produce even more hamburgers.

A lesser known fact about global warming is that the methane gas emitted by the flatulence of cattle contributes more to global warming than the exhaust emissions of all the automobiles on earth. We create chronic situations that would never exist naturally.

In the next fifty years climate changes are expected to kill off ten per cent of animal and plant life. This decimation would mean the loss of more than a million species.

A vast percentage of our drugs and medicines are made up from plant life. In destroying the rain forests, we are destroying our capability to discover future life saving drugs and medicines. This is yet another part of the lunatic price we pay for junk food.

Fast food companies face legal battles and vast compensation claims. Tobacco companies once had their heads as deep in the sand as the fast food companies do now, but that did not stop them from eventually paying out over two hundred and fifty billion dollars in compensation with many more payments still to be made.

Over one hundred and seventeen billion dollars was the estimated medical cost of obesity, last year in the U.S.

Modern science is starting to prove that food manufacturers and the doyens of fast food have a lot to answer for. At some point the food manufacturers made the mistake of believing their own advertising, at a disastrous cost to all of us.

"There are only two things our customers have,
time and money, and they don't like spending either of them,
so we have to sell them their hamburgers quickly."
- James McLamore   Founder of Burger King.

Easily Influenced

If you were asked to identify one of the main influences on children to eat a bad diet, where would you look? As children are easily influenced you might look for the worlds largest 'toy distributor'. You would be looking for a company whose rise, in the last forty years, has coincided with the onset of obesity in adults and children. It might be a good idea to look for the world's largest user of beef. Maybe you would look on your local High Street, where you will find the largest brand name in the world that spends over two billion pounds a year on advertising. If you were to look down your local High Street on October 16th you might well see a demonstration by Greenpeace outside the premises you are looking for. Greenpeace have been holding a World Day of Action against McDonalds, on that date, since the mid 1980's.

McDonalds are famous for children's birthday parties. Indeed, if you were to insist that your children cannot go to their friend's birthday party, simply because you do not want them influenced into eating junk food – what kind of killjoy would you be labelled as?

The party looked as if it might be coming to an end for McDonalds in 2003 when their expansion started to slow and they shut over 100 stores in ten countries. This of course left thirty thousand McDonalds stores still selling junk food.

McDonalds shares fell sharply on Christmas Eve 2003 in line with the rest of shares traded connected with the 100 billion dollar American beef industry. The effect of one cow contracting BSE, mad cow disease, caused an overall drop of 3.4 billion dollars in one day.

In 1955 when Ray Croc opened his first hamburger joint in Illinois, he would have had little idea of the harmful effects of junk food, or that one-day, future customers would be suing his company for the harm done to them by eating it.

John Banzhaf, Professor of law at George Washington Law School has said that, *"Companies selling food high in fat and sugar are deeply vulnerable to litigation."* In 2003 Prof. Banzhaf wrote to some of the world's foremost fast food outlets warning them of possible litigation. Among those he wrote to were: McDonalds, Burger King, Kentucky Fried Chicken and Pizza Hut.

Cause and Effect

The study of indigenous populations past and present gives us the answers to the effects of diet on our health and longevity. The evidence of what constitutes a healthy diet is blatant.

The argument that ethnic groups are physiologically different holds no sway. Change the diet of any ethnic group to one of refined and junk food and they gain weight and start to develop the same catalogue of illnesses: Heart-disease, cancer, kidney complaints and a myriad of attendant medical problems. (On page 49 there is a reference that proves, through DNA, that one small community in Africa fathered the entire human race.)

There are an estimated 176 million diabetics in the world; 140 million of these cases are directly related to obesity. The escalating diabetes statistics parallel the opening of fast food outlets, selling junk food to hitherto healthy populations.

When the multinationals export a diet of refined and junk food to the rest of the world, they make a double profit – firstly the profit on the food and secondly the profit on the drugs to counteract the damage this *food* creates.

Why are people so susceptible to junk food? Opioids are the answer. Overdosing on fat and sugar produces opioids, chemicals that change brain structure and trigger hormonal changes. The fat and sugar in junk food is so highly concentrated that it overwhelms the brains receptors.

The easiest way for a junk-food junkie to wean himself off a diet that brings obesity, illness and death is to give up junk food completely. There is no acceptable minimal amount that can be eaten of this so-called *food*. One burger and a shake contain such a highly concentrated overdose of fat and sugar that it has the same effect on the brain as a power surge would have on a computer. Junk food has to be completely avoided.

The only way to sate our core cravings for fat, sugar and salt is with natural unadulterated food that is eaten in human proportions.

" By stimulating the release of natural opioids in the brain, sugar and fat could have a similar effect to addictive drugs such as heroin."
- John Hoebel   Psychologist, Princeton University.

In 1981 Canadian, Professor David Jenkins developed the Glycaemic Index. Which is, quite simply, a ranking of foods from 0 to 100 that tells us just how quickly each specific food raises our blood sugar (glucose) levels.

There is no need for the glycaemic value of food to add any confusion to what you should or should not eat.

Knowing about the kind of energy surge that each carbohydrate delivers is invaluable to diabetics who need to avoid peaks in their blood sugar and to maintain equilibrium; they are best suited to low glycaemic foods.

Endurance athletes will eat low glycaemic food prior to exercising, and replenish the much-needed carbohydrates to their body, during and after the event by eating higher glycaemic food.

Many processed *foods*, which are highly glycaemic, such as manufactured breakfast foods, biscuits, cakes, white bread, white rice, chocolate bars and fizzy drinks are not on your agenda anyway. Just regard them as non-foods.

Virtually all manufactured breakfast *foods* are highly glycaemic including Corn Flakes, which are possibly the most popular. Children who eat these cereals for breakfast become hungry before lunchtime and are more prone to snacking on junk food.

There are a few vegetables that have been measured as highly glycaemic, but these were measured under laboratory conditions singly and not in conjunction with other foods; the body's metabolism reacts to the composition of a meal in its entirety.

The baked potato is highly glycaemic because of its high starch content. New potatoes and boiled potatoes are much lower on the glycaemic index. Interestingly the sweet potato is a low glycaemic food. Mashing boiled potatoes together with sweet potatoes not only brings down their overall glycaemic value but also increases the amount of nutrients in your meal.

Simple changes mean you can eat the food you like and have the benefit of good nutrition. Avoiding non-foods has to be a way of life.

"A fad-free approach to long term weight loss is best and that means a diet rich in fruit, vegetables and whole grains."
- Jen Keller RD

Milk

" It is now clear enough that dairy products do not build strong bones."
- Dr. Neal Barnard M.D
President of The Physicians Committee for Responsible Medicine.

Milk is <u>not</u> a natural food for human beings; it is the natural food for calves until they are ready to start eating grass. The calcium in dairy foods is negated before it reaches your bones. Cow's milk has three hundred times more casein than human milk. Dairy foods are rich in protein that acidifies the blood, to neutralise this acidity your body uses calcium. If the calcium content in the dairy food is not substantial enough to perform this neutralisation your body will leech calcium from your bones to perform this task.

The American Institute for Cancer Research have produced evidence that diets high in dairy foods increase the risk of prostate and kidney cancer. Countries with the highest intake of dairy food have the highest incidence of osteoporosis. Exercise and vitamin D are essential to build and maintain strong and healthy bones. Vitamin D is created when we expose ourselves to sunlight. A thirty minute walk in daylight four or five times a week will maintain your bone mass. Weight bearing exercises are essential for strong and healthy bones.

Consumers have been bombarded with milk propaganda and brainwashed into believing that milk is a wonder food. A glass of milk contains 116gm of calcium, fill the same glass with spears of broccoli and you have fifty per cent more calcium – this calcium is more easily absorbed and not negated by the blood-acidifying protein found in milk. Cow's milk has absolutely no goodness that we cannot find elsewhere without its side effects. What it does have are the hormones fed to the cows and the antibiotics used to treat bovine diseases. The food fed to these animals has to be suspect after BSE, mad cow disease epidemics. We have no reason to be part of such a volatile food chain!

" I do not like broccoli, and I haven't liked it since I was a kid and my mother made me eat it. And I'm President of the United States and I'm not going to eat any more broccoli."
- George Bush

Thirty percent of all people tested for allergies are allergic to dairy food. This statistic is less startling when you realise the more fortunate dairy cows eat grass treated with pesticides, and the less fortunate eat food pellets which could contain anything that will artificially increase the milk yield. Any medication these animals are treated with, such as antibiotics and steroids, find their way into our system. Milk finds its way into many foods, if the ingredients on the packet contain: caseinate, lactose or whey, they are milk derivatives.

If you were to watch a television programme that advocated giraffe's milk being fed to goats you would immediately realise you were watching a comedy. Mammals' milk is specific to its offspring, it is not transferable, the constituents of a mother's milk subtly changes from week to week to mirror the babies dietary needs through its early development. Once weaned all mammals including humans have no need for milk or its products.

In the past twenty years there have been instances of salmonella in chocolate and cheese, lysteria in soft cheese, and botulism in yoghurt. Botulism is usually associated with sausages where it incubates within the sausage skin.

All these infections are life threatening and in the above instances people have actually died.

Herbivores in the wild live on grass. But in the last few years man, in the interest of increased financial profit, decided to turn herbivores into cannibals, with the disastrous result of creating BSE, mad cow disease. We are only just beginning to find out how fragile our ecology is. It would be a mistake to think that we are getting away with murder when eating these animal products. Creutzfeldt Jakob disease has already made its way from animals to man through the food chain; afflicting 130 people in Great Britain; the few horrendous deaths it has caused could easily become many.

Due to BSE, the American Red Cross will not accept blood transfusions from anyone who lived in the U.K from 1980 to date. This graphically illustrates just how dangerous the effects of eating meat are perceived to be.

" Every human being is the author of his own health or disease."
                                                    - Sivananda

Food Poisoning

The guideline for restaurants serving eggs is to cook them well; the yolk of a fried egg should be cooked until solid. This will not remove the cholesterol content but it will kill any salmonella that the eggs might contain, although there is one strain of salmonella that can remain in eggs even after cooking.

There is a more interesting question than, why did the chicken cross the road? How did the salmonella get into the egg? Profit is the answer! Egg producers realised they were wasting a *fine* source of protein which could be fed to battery hens, this protein being their own offspring.

Man, once again, was willing to ignore the simple rules of nature and use cannibalism to enhance the hallowed bottom line. Hundreds of thousands of male chicks were gassed, pulverised and turned into feed then fed to their mothers. This horror story is part of the recent history of our food chain.

Although mass immunisation of chickens has brought the incidence of salmonella down, it has also ensured that further antibiotics have found their way into the food chain. Four hundred tons of chicken a year is consumed in the United Kingdom and over one hundred and eighty tons are infected with campylobacter, a food poisoning as virulent as salmonella. Over forty-five percent of all chicken sold in the U.K are infected with campylobacter. Campylobacter is regarded as the new bug on the block and scientists have not yet found an answer to it.

One in every eight people were infected with food poisoning in the United Kingdom in 2003 this does not take into account the many cases which go unreported. Deaths by food poisoning in 2003 of four hundred and eighty people are recognised as an underestimate.

One in three people who survive E.coli go onto die of renal disease. Other hidden, long-term effects of an assortment of food poisoning will only be known in the fullness of time. The dynamic of toxicity is subtle.

" Health is not valued until sickness comes"
- Dr. Thomas Fuller

Sugar

Now for the second villain of the piece Sugar! The case against sugar could not have been put more succinctly than by John Yudkin, in his enlightening book: Pure, White and Deadly:

" *If only a small fraction of what is already known about sugar were to be revealed in relation to any other material used as a food additive, that material would be promptly banned.*"

Any food with a refined sugar content is not a viable food to eat. It's that simple! Brown sugar is as deadly as white. In order to metabolise refined sugar your body depletes its stocks of chromium. One of the symptoms of chromium deficiency is lowered metabolism leading to weight gain. Whereas when you derive your sugar from fresh fruit it contains enough trace elements to ensure that metabolic equilibrium is maintained.

A 380mi. bottle of Lucozade sold as a *sports drink* contains over 20 level teaspoons of sugar. A 750g box of Kellogg's Special K contains over a quarter of a pound of sugar. This cereal is promoted to attract slimmers as it is advertised as low in fat.

Food or drink containing a high concentration of sugar is an anathema to the body. Sugar has many aliases: dextrose, corn- syrup, fructose, lactose, maltose, sucrose, molasses, galactose, levulose and sorghum. It is up to you to check the ingredients of the food you buy. Sugar has no nutritional value.

Sugar substitutes are mainly chemical and once they are in your body their chemical structure changes. Aspartame found in most *diet* drinks changes to formaldehyde. Yes! The very same formaldehyde used for embalming bodies. (Smoking also produces formaldehyde in the body.) In 1996 the American Association for Neuropathologists claimed there was a link between its use and a ten per cent rise in brain tumours in the 1980's.

Aspartame has no nutritional value and has been found to cause cancer in rats. Because of its easy availability to the very young, if only one percent of its detractors are correct, it is one of the most dangerous food additives. Sugar substitutes have a notorious history; in the amendment to the Pure Food Law 1913 it stated that Saccharine was:

'*A deleterious ingredient lowering the quality of food into which it is put.*'

31

Soft drinks should not be part of your diet, regardless if they're sugar filled or have the word *diet* clearly marked on them, as *diet* drinks contain artificial sweeteners that, although calorie free, will stimulate your craving for other sweet food.

To find out the calorific value of a 330ml can of Pepsi the U.K's biggest selling soft drink, you need to telephone the manufacturer, as it is not marked on the can. On phoning them they will tell you it contains 155 calories (about 12 level teaspoons of sugar). Coca Cola does not list the amount of calories on their cans either, but they will tell you that a regular can contains 142 calories (about 11 level teaspoons of sugar). From its very outset the Coca Cola Company has regarded its ingredients as top secret, but it is no secret that both Pepsi and Coca Cola, two of the most advertised products on earth, contain the drug caffeine. Caffeine is used in the manufacture of headache pills and has many other medical uses where it is prescribed in exact doses. What place has it in a drink sold to children?

How soft is a soft drink? On average Cola drinks contain half the caffeine content of a regular cup of coffee. The word *soft* in this instance must challenge for the position of the greatest misnomer of all time. It has to be accepted that a large carton of Cola is the most common accompaniment to a junk food meal, but why would anyone want to give their child a large dose of a drug, without a valid medical reason.

Many other *soft* drinks apart from Cola contain the drug caffeine and children drink them freely in copious amounts. It should come as no surprise that the potent mix of caffeine and sugar or sugar substitutes make children hyperactive. We are all aware of the effects of coffee on our own systems. The fully developed brains and bodies of adults can barely cope with this drug's onslaught and children have much less resistance. Seventy-five percent of delinquents were hyperactive as children. Children prone to hyperactivity have such a low tolerance to caffeine that even smaller amounts found in chocolate have a detrimental effect on them. Why endanger a child's health and future because of intense advertising pressure?

" Many a small thing has been made large by the right kind of advertising "
- Mark Twain.

Caffeine

Most of us have the good sense to limit our consumption of coffee and tea, as we have suffered the effects of overindulgence. Once again, much as with sugar, we get a high followed by a low. Coffee addicts can drink as much as eight or ten cups a day drinking more and more in an effort to recreate the original high they experienced, but as the body's tolerance to the drug is increased, that original high becomes less attainable. People under the influence of any addictive substance always perceive the *benefits* to be far greater than they are.

Caffeine is a stimulant to the central nervous system it raises the blood pressure and substantially increases cholesterol while obstructing the body's absorption of iron and zinc. Anyone drinking a substantial amount of caffeine filled drinks should cut down slowly, as they will suffer withdrawal symptoms.

Coffee is the second largest traded commodity in the world, coming second to oil. Although coffee consumption has fallen since the 1960's, its dramatic rise in price has insured its position at the top end of traded commodities. The fall of coffee consumption has not lowered the amount of caffeine consumed; the rise in the sale of *soft* drinks containing caffeine has tripled in the last forty years. The U.S. Market for *diet* drinks alone is three and a half billion dollars a year.

One of the least acknowledged ironies of the last hundred years involves two polarising events. More was discovered about the nutrients in food than had ever been known, while the mass production of food robbed us of those nutrients.

We place our trust in brand names, somehow believing that if a company is large enough it has to be trusted. So far, no company can claim to have enhanced the original nutritional value of any food. They take the basic material and make less of it. They spend fortunes of your money on research of how to get more money from you by concocting some new addictive *treat*. Once concocted they spend more of your money on advertising, alerting you to its: *enhanced flavour, added vitamins and amazing nutritional value.*

" Advertising is the cheapest way of selling goods,
even if the goods are worthless." - Sinclair Lewis.

Salt

The cynical saga of the Emperor's New Clothes is played out every time a new product is launched. If they get the balance of salt, sugar, fat and additives just right they could be onto a winner. A product the public cannot get enough of - a product destined to gain its market share.

The U.K government wants the amount of salt in food reduced but this has to be achieved slowly because the consumer has to be weaned off the extraordinary amount of salt finding its way into package foods. Salt is a flavour enhancer; it also disguises the amount of sugar in a product. If you were to taste something sickly sweet you would immediately reject it. This is not the case when sweetness is masked with salt. You end up eating abnormal amounts of both salt and sugar. We need salt in our diet, it is important, but only in very minimal amounts. Over eighty per cent of the salt in our diets comes from manufactured food, because the quantity is disguised, many of us are addicted to salt without even knowing it. A high salt intake is directly linked to strokes, heart attacks and stomach cancer. There are currently 878,000 heart failure patients a year in the United Kingdom.

A leading Japanese researcher Dr. Shoichiro Tsugane who studied 40,000 people over 10 years found that people eating double their recommended salt intake, doubled their chances of contracting stomach cancer. Cancer Research U.K verifies these findings.

The recommended amount of salt intake is 5g per day for an adult which is about one level teaspoonful with the amount decreasing substantially for children under ten. A portion of beans on toast contains an adult's complete salt intake for the day. A portion of Pizza contains virtually two days recommended salt intake for an adult. These foods are children's favourites, delivering double and quadruple their recommended daily salt intake in just one meal. Children eat packets of salt laden crisps that in turn make them thirsty for sugar filled drinks, doubly boosting food manufacturers profits. Salt is often disguised by being listed as sodium. Salt content is sodium multiplied by 2.5.

" Cornflakes are as salty as seawater"
- Professor G. Macgregor, St. Georges Hospital. U.K

The mass production of food is one of the biggest businesses on the planet. Eye catching packaging makes for instant attraction; preservatives make for a longer shelf life. You set out to buy some food and end up buying a package deal. For busy people who believe that they do not have the time to prepare fresh food, convenience food is seductive. It looks good and saves precious time. We could make use of that hackneyed old saying: *"It's the greatest invention since sliced bread!"*

Was sliced bread such a great invention? It's definitely big business. At its peak fifty million white sliced loaves were consumed per week in the U.K. alone, each containing over twenty additives including chalk and bleach. It was recently reported in the U.K. press that 3-MCPD the cancer causing carcinogenic was recently found in Mothers Pride bread, one of the U.K's top selling brands. This cancer-causing chemical finds its way into many foods. Thirty percent of manufactured foods tested at random were found to contain it.

A couple of slices of toast covered in butter, filled with saturated fat and some marmalade full of white sugar; is the *perfect* finale to an English breakfast, already overflowing with saturated fat quickly converted to cholesterol.

If you want some indication of the struggle your digestive system has to undergo when eating a baguette, the bread in vogue at the moment, remove the soft white bread from the centre of the baguette and knead it for a few seconds in the palm of your hand. Do you really think your digestive system could do anything useful with this glutinous mass? Instead of this food giving you energy, it saps you of it, as your digestive system tries to cope with something alien to it.

More and more of the population are becoming intolerant to wheat! Food that, in its unadulterated state, once gave them energy now depletes their strength. Our bodies are in rebellion against a barrage of refined food and carcinogenic chemicals. In the realm of *staple* foods: food intolerance to wheat is closely followed by food intolerance to milk.

" Thirty thousand lives are lost in Britain every year because of weight related diseases."
- Dr. John Reid   U.K. Health Secretary.

Food Intolerance

Although only three per cent of adults and six per cent of children in the U.K are affected by food allergies, half of the population are affected by food intolerance.

The unlucky few who are allergic to certain foods have to be continuously on guard. One of the most dangerous allergies is to peanuts, as it can bring about anaphylaxis, which can be fatal. Fortunately these extreme allergic reactions are very rare.

Constant overexposure to a particular food breaks down the ability to tolerate it. It is not surprising that a constant diet of sandwiches made up of white bread would eventually render a vast percentage of those who eat them intolerant to wheat. Wheat finds its way into countless foods. Eventually less and less of the offending food has the same adverse reaction and then has to be avoided completely.

Milk products take a close second place in the list of foods that we are intolerant to, but as already explained; we should never have been eating milk products to begin with. Once past the age of three the human body ceases to produce rennin and lactase, the enzymes that digest milk.

The main symptoms manifested by food intolerance are lethargy, depression, bloating, headaches, migraines, asthma and skin problems.

Many people who are intolerant to a particular food find themselves drawn to eating more and more of it, until the very food that once satisfied them leaves them feeling ill.

Reactions to allergenic foods can cause changes in the blood's chemistry, sometimes even leading to mental disorders.

The human body is naturally intolerant to alcohol and caffeine, and we can easily develop a craving for them, in much the same way as we develop a craving for foods we are intolerant to. The perversity of the situation is frustrating, but it can be easily rectified.

Before going on a diet, a food intolerance test makes sense. Your doctor can easily refer you for an allergy and intolerance test, which is simple and painless.

" When meditating over a disease, I never think of finding a remedy for it, but, instead, a means of preventing it. – Louis Pasteur.

Dangerous Ingredients

The water biscuit is probably the most innocuous of the hundreds of different varieties of biscuit on supermarket shelves.

Here are the ingredients of a simple water biscuit: wheat-flour, vegetable and hydrogenated vegetable oil, raising agent: sodium hydrogen carbonate, salt and glucose syrup.

Hydrogenated vegetable oil is found in most biscuits and breakfast cereals. Hydrogenation takes a natural product and turns it into something lethal. Hydrogenation is a chemical process that converts polyunsaturated fats into trans fatty acids. Essentially, vegetable fat is made solid by adding hydrogen atoms. Be assured this transformation is not for the benefit of your health. This process is undertaken to create texture and ensure the shelf life of biscuits and breakfast cereals. Innocuous oils are turned into substances that endanger your heart for the benefit of their texture and sell-by date.

Most margarine has undergone hydrogenation, which hardens vegetable oil until it has the consistency of butter. The change in the molecular structure of this oil has far reaching effects, when your body attempts to convert it to fuel. Apart from increasing the bad cholesterol (LDL) in your body, it reduces the good cholesterol (HDL). There are 3,500 calories in a pound of human bodyweight, approximately the same amount of calories as in a pound of Margarine.

Nature got it right to begin with! The manipulation of food is invariably to its detriment. If food contains hydrogenated oil it should not be on your shopping list, regardless of the fact that it might be sold as one hundred per cent vegetable oil. Many companies are trying to replace trans fatty acids in their products, fearful of possible lawsuits in the future. Common sense tells you that there is no tolerable level for taking toxins into your body. Zero tolerance is the only answer.

" The perils inherent in the industrialised production of food now pose perhaps the greatest threat to the health of mankind."
- Ivan Illich.

Traditional Dangers

Take unsaturated oil and heat it to a high degree and you change its molecular structure, it becomes mutagenic. Trans fatty acids begin to form; once you consume these trans fatty acids they damage the protective barrier around your cells seriously affecting your health at its most basic level. This makes fried food, especially deep-fried food, which is cooked at very high temperatures so detrimental to your wellbeing.

In the U.S.A deep-fried chicken and fries, in the U.K traditional fish and chips, attack your system at the molecular level. In essence, when you eat food that has been deep-fried a good percentage of what you are eating is toxic waste.

The deep fat fryer, heats oil to a high temperature throughout the day, constantly changing its molecular structure. Eventually, at the end of the day the oil is allowed to cool and has to be disposed of as toxic waste. If somebody offered to pay you to eat a tablespoon full of this toxic waste, you would refuse; but consider this; an hour earlier you were actually paying to eat a few tablespoonfuls of this very same oil suffused into your meal.

Once the toxic waste leaves the restaurant its life is far from over; it is sold to recyclers who add caustic soda and alcohol to it, which turns it into resaleable diesel fuel.

Great care must be taken when cooking food with oil. Stir- frying is good, as the process is fast and very little oil is needed. To roast vegetables, initially dry roast them and add olive oil in the last few minutes. Olive oil is monounsaturated and can be heated to three hundred and twenty five degrees without destroying its fatty acids.

With a little ingenuity traditional culinary effects can be recreated by using the right kind of oil in small quantities added at the right time.

Fish is an essential part of our diet, to enjoy its amazing nutritional benefits it only needs to be grilled or baked.

" There's a theory, that man evolved in areas bordering seas and lakes because fish provided material for brain development which other species lacked. So the folklore that said fish is food for the brain may be vindicated. " - Prof. A.E. Bender   University of London.

Microwaves

Any estate agent worth his sodium will tell you that if you put a decent kitchen into your home it will add value.

Once upon a time the kitchen was a topsy-turvy place where food was cooked. Today many kitchens are just a pristine investment where only the microwave and the corkscrew are used.

Dr. David Holden of Auckland, New Zealand. Has made a detailed study on the effects of microwaves on food. Dr. Holden deserves much credit for his efforts, as the multinational companies who produce microwave ovens, have vehemently defended their domain and profits in the past, with all manner of gagging orders and court injunctions. But the truth could not be suppressed forever!

Here is Dr. Holden's forthright and succinct opinion:

" Microwave cooking is one of the most important causes of ill health, it is certainly one of the most ignored.

Normal heating of food occurs when heat goes from the outside to the inside. Microwaves work just the opposite. The waves go to the inside and then move outward. The food molecules are hit by the electromagnetic radiation and forced to reverse polarity quickly. That is, the molecules start spinning. This tears them apart and sometimes rearranges them into toxic substances that cause many allergic responses. It is the friction, which produces the heat that 'cooks' the food. It is no longer 'food' – it just looks as though it is."

This has to be the ultimate description of non-food:

'It is no longer 'food' – it just looks as though it is.'

Food can be speedily cooked by: frying in a wok - which needs the smallest amount of oil, conventional roasting, or if you are cooking vegetables, use a steamer, if you haven't already got one, they are a fabulous investment. Steam heat is hotter than boiling water, so your vegetables are cooked quickly and their nutrients are not leached away into the boiled water, which is then discarded.

Another piece of kitchen equipment that is essential is a good electric blender, for making fresh soups and smoothies. Blenders do everything that expensive juicers do, with less mess and expense.

Non-Food

Breakfast foods, potato crisps and crispbreads have been found to contain 100 times the permitted amount of the cancer causing chemical Acrylamide.

Acrylamide is a cancer-causing chemical found in cooked and processed food. The higher the temperature the food reaches when being manufactured, the higher the possible content of acrylamide. The chemical acrylamide is used in papermaking. European rules relating to the amount of acrylamide allowed in food packaging are no more than ten parts per billion. Tests have shown that over one thousand parts per billion of acrylamide are present in some top brand name varieties of crisps, breakfast foods and crispbreads. There is currently no scientific way of preparing these manufactured foods without creating acrylamide. Apart from many foods being filled with preservatives, additives, salt, sugar and fat they have the carcinogen acrylamide in them. These *foods* must be avoided! They are non-foods.

When you buy food, real-food is what you want, not some adulterated product. Do not entertain non-foods.

Bearing in mind the toxicity in these products, the audacious ploy of advertising added vitamins in breakfast foods is an insult to the purchaser. Who in their right mind needs a breakfast food manufacturer to feed them half a vitamin pill?

Current legislation is about to make food labelling less ambiguous, here is the ruling on the word natural: " *Natural can only be used if the ingredients are produced by nature, not the work of man or interfered with by man and containing no artificial chemicals.*"

There are other legislative changes to be implemented in food labelling – and not a moment too soon. Pure natural food is your right.

" Do you know what breakfast cereal is made of?
It's made of all those little curly wooden shavings
you find in pencil sharpeners." – Roald Dahl.

Shelf Life

Each year in the United Kingdom, twenty five thousand tons of over five hundred diverse pesticides are sprayed onto our food. Not only are the pests removed by the pesticides they also deplete half of the calcium, potassium, iron and selenium from our fruit and vegetables. Lettuce, the food to which most dieters gravitate, was found in random government tests to have well above the allowed pesticide residue in over fifty per cent of tested crops. Lettuce had well above the average pesticide residue because of its large surface area. Pesticide residue is mainly a surface problem, rigorous washing of fruit and vegetables reduces pesticide residue dramatically.

We live in an age where science fact supersedes science fiction on a daily basis. The irradiation of food is the science of the invisible; food is exposed to gamma rays from a radioactive source, passing through the food, the rays split the DNA of the food's natural bacteria, killing the bacteria and increasing its shelf life.

The only way of knowing if fresh fruit and vegetables have been irradiated is when they give themselves away. Those strawberries that refuse to go rotten, but get a little darker each day as the few nutrients left after irradiation deplete.

The three most important things in the supermarket business as far as fresh produce is concerned are: shelf life, shelf life and shelf life.

The move towards organic food ebbs and flows as the supermarkets have an on and off love affair with the idea of promoting organic food, hopefully the organic section in your supermarket will expand with the will of consumers eager to buy organic food. Supermarkets inevitably bow to purchasing power.

" *Food one assumes provides nourishment, but Americans eat it*
fully aware that small amounts of poison have been added
to improve its appearance and delay putrefaction."
- John Cage

In the U.K. during the Second World War, to economise on fuel and labour, a system called zoning was used to ensure that commodities and food did not travel a greater distance than they needed to. The U.K was split up into zones and each zone became self-sufficient. We now employ a system that is the exact opposite.

Apples travel over ten thousand miles from the U.S.A to the U.K. Research show that the further fruit and vegetables travel the more their vitamins and minerals are depleted. Apples that were once plentiful in the U.K are now quite rare. You will rarely see Ribston Pippins, D'arcy Spice, Lord Lambournes, Blenheim Orange, Eccleston Orange or Crispins just to name a few of the wonderful apples we have been denied because they are not regarded as profitable enough; as they have a lower yield than the few varieties forced upon us by the supermarkets.

In the last twenty-five years, half of the apple orchards in the U.K have disappeared, along with dozens of different varieties of apples. Image obsession even affects apples. European standards decree that if an apple is not the perfect shape it cannot be eaten and enjoyed, no matter how fresh and wholesome it might be.

Notwithstanding the diminution of choice, there is a cost to the environment in greenhouse emissions and a cost to the consumer, who pays dearly for jet fuel, to bring food that once grew abundantly in their backyard.

The National Farmer's Union reported that virtually seventy-five percent of what we pay for food in the supermarket is made up of: transport, packaging, processing, advertising and a massive mark-up that can be as high as fifty percent. In some chronic instances the grower gets just one percent of what we pay for fruit at the checkout.

We are being overcharged and we are unwittingly exploiting people in the third world at the same time. We are not helpless; by simply changing our diet we can change the situation.

The Food Standards Association maintain that fresh vegetables, which undergo long refrigerated journeys, do not retain their nutrients as much as frozen vegetables.

"You cannot sell a blemished apple in the supermarket,
you can sell a tasteless one provided its shiny, smooth,
even, uniform and bright."   - Elspeth Huxley

Emotional Eating

With the exception of politicians there are few people who have not gone through periods of low self-esteem in their lives. Questioning our self worth is a part of being human. We want to do our best and be our best, and it is all too easy to fall short of our own expectations.

Eating as a consolation when we are at a low ebb, or when things go wrong, is a common scenario but attempting to fill an emotional void with food is impossible. You cannot eat your way out of trouble.

In the first instance, the overweight person has to do some soul searching to determine if their weight problem is due to emotional eating, a faulty diet due to lack of knowledge about nutrition, or in very rare cases, a physiological problem. A combination of these problems is of course more difficult to determine.

Although many pundits and gurus are willing to give glib answers to emotional eating problems, nobody can experience the world from the unique perspective of the person caught in the web of their own thinking process.

Many people become depressed simply because they are overweight and end up eating more to comfort themselves for feeling wretched; setting up a vicious circle to which the only means of escape they can perceive is yo-yo dieting, which in turn compounds their situation. This situation can only be overcome by eating real-food in human proportions and exercising moderately on a regular basis.

Deep-seated emotional problems, many of which stem back to childhood, invariably need professional help. According to the NSPCC, at this very moment in the United Kingdom 34,000 children are suffering abuse. They need help now! They will also need help in the future as, unfortunately they will be part of our next generation of people with serious eating disorders as fifty percent of bulimics suffered sexual abuse as children.

"Eating disorders whether Anorexia or Bulimia, show how individuals can turn the nourishment of the body into a painful attack on themselves, and they have at the core, a far deeper problem than vanity." - Diana Princess of Wales

Image obsession is forced upon us; you only have to look through the pages of any magazine to find it filled with amazingly svelte, airbrushed, beautiful people. These beautiful people hardly represent a minute percentage of what people actually look like in the real world; but to the suggestible the damage is done.

It is far more dangerous to be seven pounds underweight than fourteen pounds overweight. This message is virtually impossible to convey to anybody suffering from anorexia or bulimia; eating disorders at the other end of the spectrum to obesity.

Calorie counting diets can cause havoc to anyone with an obsessive personality. Human beings by their very nature are spontaneous; if we were only surrounded by natural nourishing food as opposed to manufactured, processed and junk food, the possibility that we might derive more energy from one food or another would not only be boring, it would be totally irrelevant. All that needs to be understood is how to eat nourishing food in human proportions.

The law of thermodynamics; which states that energy cannot disappear or be created from nothing, is fundamental as far as physics are concerned, but it is a dangerous concept in the hands of a vulnerable anorexic or bulimic girl who is willing to take calorie counting to its abysmal extreme.

A recent study found that regularly eating peanuts increases the metabolism, an interesting scenario, when the fuel can change the dynamic of the engine. It just so happens that all calories are not created equal. In another study conducted at the City of Hope National Medical Centre in California it was found that two controlled groups of people, eating exactly the same amount of restricted calories, did not have the same weight loss. One group lost considerably more, as part of their calorie intake was made up of almonds. It was speculated that the fibre of the nut compromised the absorption of its fat. This of course establishes a precedent as far as calories are concerned. Counting calories would only work if all calories were equal; if, as it seems, they are not, a lot of obsessive calorie counters will have to totally rethink their strategy.

"Beautiful young people are accidents of nature,
but beautiful old people are a work of art." – Eleanor Roosevelt.

44

Protein

All proteins are made up of amino acids of which there are twenty-four. They are prime energy sources; they help break down fat for energy. Apart from improving mental alertness, and lifting mood they promote resistance to disease and quicken reflexes.

The building blocks of protein amino acids strengthen the body's connective tissues preventing injury.

Interacting with each other, the twenty-four known amino acids continuously repair and replicate every fibre of the human body. Although the body can produce sixteen of these amino acids, the other eight, called essential, are found in food.

To perform all the tasks needed to repair and maintain your body, billions of combinations have to be produced using these twenty-four initial building blocks.

The following is a minute percentage of the functions that the essential amino acids derived from food perform:

Leucine plus Isoleucine: increase mental alertness.

Lysine: helps form collagen, absorb calcium, produces antibodies, hormones and enzymes. A deficiency results in fatigue, irritability and a lack of concentration.

Methionine: lowers cholesterol and protects the kidneys. Prevents disorders of the hair, skin and nails and promotes hair growth.

Phenylalanine: produces norepinephrine the chemical that transmits signals between nerve cells and the brain. Reduces hunger pains, maintains alertness, improves memory and is a natural antidepressant.

Threopnine: regulates metabolism and aids digestion and is instrumental in creating collagen, elastin and enamel protein.

Tryptophan: alleviates insomnia, reduces the risk of artery and heart spasms. In conjunction with lysine reduces cholesterol.

Valine: promotes mental energy and muscle coordination.

An imbalance of amino acids attacks the basic structure of mind and body. Alcohol and drugs throw your brain's receptors into chaos attacking the epicentre of your existence.

" Change your thoughts and you change your world!"
        - Norman Vincent Peale

Over ten million people in the USA are affected by alcohol abuse. The havoc alcohol causes to the body is mirrored by the effect it has on society, you only have to stumble across a drunk on the sidewalk to realise where alcohol can ultimately lead.

Alcohol destroys families. It is a long and tortuous road on the way to rock bottom, and it makes no sense why rock bottom has to be achieved before people decide to make a change. This notion that rock bottom is the pivotal moment to induce change needs serious rethinking.

You will often hear the case made, that one or two glasses of red wine a day are beneficial. It is far more beneficial to eat red or black grapes each day, as the goodness you seek is in their skins, they contain resveratrol an anti-blood clotting agent. This way you get the full benefit of the upside without the downside.

Alcohol hits the brain like a sledgehammer - you forget your worries and lose your inhibitions, and leave yourself vulnerable to every mishap imaginable. While alcohol assails your brain it depletes your body of its nutrients. It has ruined countless brilliant careers and stopped even more careers from ever getting started.

Alcohol robs people of their personality! Alcohol assails the brains chemistry and sets up a dependency; just as a virus takes hold, alcohol takes hold. Once alcohol sets up residence in the body, it proceeds to destroy it.

Alcohol and drugs affect the neurotransmitters of the brain creating an imbalance in the levels of our amino acids; we then make the futile attempt of trying to rebalance these amino acids, by taking more of the very thing that caused the imbalance. Although simplistic this is the basis of addiction.

One of the most recent therapies for treating addiction to alcohol and drugs involves taking amino acids, which reinstate the status quo. Once reinstated, a natural diet containing all the nutrients needed to ensure you have balanced levels of amino acids is all that is needed to regain physiological equilibrium. With the fog lifted the chances of addressing the psychological problems at the root cause are enhanced.

" It is no measure of health to be well adjusted
to a profoundly sick society. "   - Krishnamurti.

Fourteen million people a year are treated for depression in the United States. Eighty percent of those that seek treatment are prescribed anti-depressants. Your estimate is as good as mine as to how many million people do not seek treatment and suffer in silence or turn to drink.

Carl Jung was indirectly responsible for the inception of Alcoholics Anonymous. A man approached Jung seeking help with a drinking problem. Jung told the man that he knew of no cure but believed that the crux of the problem was a lack of spirituality and that was the reason drinkers consumed alcohol. Jung recommended that the man should take up religion and go to church. The man taking Jung's advice took up religion and managed to give up drink.

A few years later, another man with the same problem approached Jung. Aware that religion had apparently worked for the first man, Jung put the two men in touch with each other.

The two men proceeded to go to church together and the second man gave up drink. The two men then found that just talking about their problems with each other kept them sober, without the help of organised religion. These two men formed the first enclave of Alcoholics Anonymous. This in effect, was the birth of group therapy.

Millions of people throughout the world are attempting to fill emotional voids with: food, alcohol and drugs. We cannot exist in a vacuum and we cannot always solve all of our problems ourselves. Sometimes we need to help each other. And it is best to take action long before rock bottom is even contemplated.

When the problem is serious, action must be taken quickly. Both Alcoholics Anonymous and Overeaters Anonymous are run voluntarily, there is no charge. Compassion and understanding is what underpins recovery – The credo of, *"One day at a time"* has helped millions of people throughout the world to lead happy and fulfilled lives. AA and OA have branches everywhere and are in the phone book. Addiction is an illness; it makes the strong vulnerable, robbing them of their health and dignity. AA and OA do not suit everybody, but one visit to a meeting might help point in the right direction.

" We cannot change anything unless we accept it,
Condemnation does not liberate it oppresses." - Carl Jung

The Bigger Picture

It is fashionable these days to talk of the 'bigger picture' unfortunately the bigger picture is far from flattering. As a growing number of people die of obesity in the western world, twenty four thousand people a day, three quarters of them children, die of starvation in the third world. Are the obese of the western world gluttons or baffled victims of circumstance?

It takes ten pounds of grain to produce one pound of meat. Notwithstanding the slaughter of the animals, it is hard to justify eating meat when you realise that, if the western world gave up eating meat, the third world could be fed without the production of an extra pound of grain. In a year, one acre of land produces nine times the potato protein as beef protein. Soya beans produce an even higher yield of high quality protein per acre. Soya contains ten times the protein of milk.

When we eat meat we harm far more than ourselves. If by eating a healthier diet we could save just one child on the other side of the planet, why would we need to think twice about it?

Thirteen million children a year die of hunger and malnutrition. Future generations will look back on us and wonder why we could not make simple changes when faced with blatant facts. We are suffering the disastrous results of apathy.

The initial changes, which need to be made, do not need to be enforced by any government, if we all decided tomorrow to eat a healthier diet; the changes would start to occur naturally and the bigger picture would come sharply into focus.

Poverty engenders malnutrition, which breeds diseases such as tuberculosis, which travels at the speed of a jet plane from the heart of Africa to the heart of London.

In 2002, three thousand people contracted tuberculosis, a disease thought of as a thing of the past because of medical advances. It is estimated that if the current trend in tuberculosis continues, fifty per cent of the world's population will have contracted it by 2010.

" The war against hunger is truly mankind's war of liberation"
- John F Kennedy

DNA has proved that the complete human population originated from the Bushmen of the Kalahari. Over the last twenty-five thousand years, our ancestors literally walked out of Africa.

Amazingly the San Bushmen who remained in the Kalahari Desert continued to live as hunter-gatherers until Dutch and German colonialists, their *civilised* descendants, returned in the last three hundred years to decimate them and destroy their culture.

Would it have made any difference to these colonialists had they realised that these were the living remnants of their ancestors, instead of some sub-species of humans that, they assumed, they had just happened upon? Probably not, when you realise that the surface of the land they inhabited was then covered in diamonds.

The diamonds are now locked safely in vaults and safe-deposits throughout the western world while the San people, the living remnant of our ancestors, are dispossessed. Traumatised by their treatment, their complete history, passed orally from one generation to another in stories and song, is virtually obliterated. An important part of our history was wantonly destroyed.

These people are the oldest genetic stock of contemporary humanity, and only 110,000 of them survive, living in poverty. Instead of being revered as a living part of our ancestry they are rejected and contemplate extinction. Chances are they will be *exploited* yet again for whatever else geneticists might be able to determine for our benefit.

The San people, through DNA, are living proof of Darwin's theory of evolution. Ethnic differences are intrinsically due to our adapting to our surroundings and our gene pool being restricted to those in close proximity to us. We are all made of the same basic material.

The human race is one family; we all have a vested interest in each other. You are only as strong as the weakest immune system of any one of six billion of your fellow men. Poverty and poor hygiene engender disease and pandemics know no barrier. Viruses strike the rich as easily as the poor. Our greatest investment is ensuring that our extended family, our fellow men, are well fed and healthy. This protects our immediate family. Apathy could easily destroy us!

"When perfect order prevails the world is like a home shared by all."
                                                        - Confucious

A Pandemic Waiting to Happen

The most devastating epidemic in human history, the 1918 influenza pandemic killed more people than died in the First World War. It is estimated that between twenty-five and fifty million people died. The true figure will remain unknown as China one of the greatest areas of devastation held no official records.

It was believed at the time that the epidemic started in Southern China - an area now recognised as the epicentre of influenza epidemics.

In 2003 the deadly Sars virus, severe acute respiratory syndrome, infected four thousand people worldwide, killing over two hundred people. A catastrophe was contained by speedy medical action. But this was just a wake-up call. Scientists say that it will be particularly difficult to develop a vaccine for Sars in the future, as the virus mutates rapidly.

Sars is highly communicable, as with many variants of influenza it originates in poultry and wildlife and is easily contractible by humans. The easiest way to fight this disease would be to attack it at its very source – by bringing hygiene to China's food markets.

In Xin Yuan Market in the Guan Dong Province of Southern China, where as recently as January 2004 there was no improvement in hygiene nine months after the initial outbreak of Sars. Crates of live rats, foxes, dogs and wild cats were piled up on each other as the animals wait to be slaughtered for *food*. In this breeding ground for future epidemics, cross contamination of species; that would never usually come into close contact with each other is inevitable. Hygiene conditions could not have been worse in the fourteenth century, at time of the Bubonic Plague.

You might well be horrified that in the twenty-first century humans could possibly eat: rats, dogs and cats and you might feel affronted, but if you happen to be a poultry and meat eater, you can be sure that your double standards would soon be pointed out to you. The Chinese are well aware of our shortcomings in the west, which include the horrific battery farming of poultry.

" The only way to live is to let live."
- Mahatma Gandhi.

Spiritual Equation

"If eating meat is not justifiable, how can we justify eating fish?" Eventually this question is always asked; here is a simple scenario that illustrates the basic spiritual level of the equation.

Let's assume you go to the cinema to see an adult film, containing the amount of violence expected of this kind of film.

Before the main feature, there is a short film that begins with a fishing trawler leaving the coastline, in the light of a brilliant sunrise. There are various shots of fisherman netting the shimmering catch in the early morning light. The next shot is of a Mediterranean port. People at the quayside are buying fish and the scene's calming effect promotes the audience to start thinking about holidaymaking. There is an air of relaxation throughout the auditorium.

The next shot is of some cows in a field, they are being pushed through a narrow gateway, into an abattoir, there's a sweeping shot of blood being hosed down a drain, there's the screeching of frightened animals. There are close-ups of fear in their eyes.

There is an immediate change of atmosphere; some people in the audience look away as the film becomes more graphic, showing close-up after close-up of cows' throats being cut. A woman in the audience screams, a man shouts out in disgust.

There are shots of ……… … …I'll spare you the details.

The reaction to watching this film proves nothing that we did not already know about ourselves. We are deeply affected by the suffering and death of any sentient being. This is the quality that makes us so unique!

We feel an affinity with dolphins and whales, the mammals of the sea, we protect them; we inherently see shoals of fish quite differently. Our instincts and reactions supply us with the answer.

" You cannot teach a man anything,
you can only help him to find it within himself."
- Galileo

Water

Often when we think we are hungry, we are actually only thirsty. This is a common misapprehension that we make much of the time.

The human being is seventy percent water; the average adult is made up of approximately eighty pints of water. Every function of our body depends on us drinking water throughout the day. We need constant re-hydration. After oxygen, water is our highest priority. A loss of fifteen to twenty percent of our body's water content is life threatening. Alcohol, sugar, salt and caffeine deplete the body of water.

Our body constantly recycles its water supply - our digestive system uses gallons of recycled water to digest our food.

Wasting water is not just selfish but ultimately foolish. We turn on a tap and expect it to be there, but this is a resource we definitely do not want to take for granted.

The world consumption of water doubles every twenty years, over a billion people in thirty countries are suffering a shortage of water at this very moment. Every fifteen seconds a child dies through lack of water. We must never forget how precious water is!

Pesticides, heavy metals and mining waste contaminate rivers and reservoirs. Climate change means that underground reservoirs are being depleted without being refilled.

Our planet is seventy percent water, but only three percent of that is fresh water. Desalination of seawater on a grand scale would be an expensive process, both financially and environmentally, as it would be a project, given today's technology, which would need to involve the nuclear industry.

We each need to drink a minimum of three pints of water a day to function properly.

Detox diets that involve drinking copious amounts of water are dangerous. They can lower the serum sodium levels in the body to such an extent that we become seriously ill. When we eat and drink correctly we are in a constant state of detox. No detox diet will ever improve on the amazing detoxification system inherent in our bodies.

"How inappropriate to call this planet Earth,
when it is so clearly Ocean." - Arthur C. Clark.

Part Two
Real-Food

"To bake an apple pie from scratch,
one first has to invent the Universe."
  - Carl Sagan

A Proven Diet

The longevity of the Japanese on the Island of Okinawa is renowned. These islanders live longer than people anywhere else on earth. Their diet consists mainly of rice, vegetables, fruit and fish.

Everything came together exquisitely for these people, the location in which they evolved was bountiful with the right food. It would seem that longevity brings wisdom. Remaining faithful to a simple life, they allowed *progress* in the form of manufactured food to pass them by.

That overused cliché " *a balanced diet* " is one of the emptiest phrases in diet jargon as it is rarely explained in any detail.

To achieve the fine balance necessary - discarding certain *food* is imperative, although adding Omega oil, vegetables and fruit will help, without giving up certain food, the benefits are only partial.

Eskimos who live on a diet high in Omega-3 fatty acids have a low incidence of heart disease and cancer, but a lack of green vegetables, which contain Omega-6 fatty acids, leaves them prone to strokes and infections.

The balancing of our diets is essential and can only be achieved through a deeper understanding of the food we eat. We need to know the fundamental truth about food before we can make a judgement about what to eat. We need a deeper understanding of nutritional values.

Becoming a pesco-vegan, a fish-eating vegan, might once have seemed like a radical move, but when you weigh the consequences of not becoming a fish-eating vegan, you realise that eating meat, poultry, junk food and refined packet food - is actually the radical diet. Non-foods have been foisted on us. We have been caught up in a myth!

When a detailed analysis is made of the health of the earth's populations, a pesco-vegan diet, eaten in human proportions is without doubt the diet for health, longevity and normal weight maintenance. This is the fundamental truth about food.

> " *Whoever the father of illness might have been,*
> *its mother was poor nutrition* "
> - Japanese proverb

The Mediterranean Diet

The Mediterranean Diet covers the diet of many countries and cultures. In the landmark 'Seven Countries Study' undertaken in the 1960s, it was determined that the risk of dying of heart disease in Italy was twice as high as on the Island of Crete. The Cretans had one of the healthiest diets in the world; unfortunately, in the last forty years, tourism accompanied by pizzas, fries and junk food, infiltrated their diet and there has been a gradual deterioration in the islanders' health.

It is very sad that thousands of years of longevity in the Cretan population were traded for non-food. Our diet needs to follow the very best aspects of The Mediterranean Diet by reaching back in time to the Cretan diet of the 1960s, which relied on eating fish regularly.

The Omega-3 fatty acids found in fish such as: mackerel, herring, sardines, pilchards, trout, anchovies and salmon are extremely beneficial to our health, and proven to be so. Unsaturated fat has the opposite effect on the body of saturated fat. It enhances life as opposed to destroying it. It rebuilds our cells.

The favourable effects of Omega-3 fatty acids are interesting. Violent offences among prisoners in Great Britain fell by forty per cent when their diet was altered to contain three servings of fish rich in Omega 3 oil per week. People suffering from depression were also found to benefit from uplift in mood when the amount of Omega 3 oil they consumed was increased.

The best fish to eat are sardines, mackerel, herring and pilchards. These fish, low in the food chain, are not contaminated with any appreciable doses of mercury and dioxins, as their life span is short.

Larger fish consume smaller fish as opposed to just algae, which along with their longer life, compounds their chemical content.

Man has been fishing for eons, a fossilised fishing-net discovered in Finland has been carbon dated as being twelve thousand years old.

" A diet of fish containing Omega-3 was essential for the necessary cerebral expansion which transformed our predecessors into Homo-sapiens. Brain capacity expanded rapidly in our prehistoric ancestors living in East Africa near large fresh water lakes. If we don't go back to our fish eating days, evolution is in danger of going into reverse."

- Professor Michael Crawford. PHD

Zen II

Any inner conflict you may have experienced in the past when trying to alter your diet is understandable. When you attempt the impossible, failure is predetermined. Your subconscious could not be fooled - it intuitively knew that something was wrong. Your inner-self was aware that you were trying to exist on sub standard fuel.

Now that you are beginning to understand the truth about food you must trust your free will implicitly. Inner transition is a gradual process that sets its own pace. There is no panic to get to where you are going, a healthier, leaner, fitter you exists in the future. Every time you set out on a twenty or thirty minute walk you are walking towards that healthier, leaner, fitter person.

You are in the position to take advantage of everything that has been discovered in the last fifty years about the goodness in real-food.

When you eat real-food, in human proportions, at regular intervals, you get a constant flow of energy. Energy powers life!

If you manage to add swimming and yoga to your exercise program, you will be on the threshold of finding peace of mind; wellbeing engenders peace of mind. Exercise is an integral part of life's equation.

You are your own guru - you don't need an intermediary to put you in touch with the power that exists within you. Every time you breathe you release that power.

You might be sitting in a traffic jam or standing in a supermarket queue – these are precious moments of your life that should not be wasted. All you need to do is straighten your spine, so that you are sitting or standing completely upright and breathe deeply and evenly.

Clearing your mind, straightening your spine and breathing deeply is how you get totally in touch with yourself. The more often you do this, the easier it is to banish stress from your life and ensure that your destiny remains in your control.

" I always looked outside myself for strength and confidence,
but it comes from within, it was there all the time."
- Anna Freud.

Simple Changes

The first battle is won in the supermarkets. Certain supermarket aisles need to become alien to you. In fact over seventy percent of the supermarket needs to become a no-go area, making shopping a speedier operation. Non-foods need to be totally avoided.

Meat, poultry and dairy foods are out. Aisles of man-made snacks and fizzy drinks are out. Virtually all manufactured and processed foods are out. Dangerous fat, sugar and salt must not get past your supermarket trolley; which is your first line of defence!

You are concentrating on fresh fruit and vegetables, fresh herbs, dried fruit and nuts, brown-rice, oatmeal, whole grain bread, rye bread, fresh fish, canned fish, dried beans, tinned beans, pulses, grains, sprouting seeds and beans etc.

Just as everything came together exquisitely for the Islanders of Okinawa, everything can just as easily come together for you. You are going to eat the most nutritious food on earth in human proportions.

Misguided notions of calorific values, that might have dogged you in the past, will eventually become a thing of the past.

Your interest is now in nutritional values. You need to become so conversant with the nutritional goodness in food, that the very thought of eating is going to make you feel good.

Within a week, your body will begin to detoxify naturally and your sense of taste will become more acute.

You are not only about to change your shape you are about to change your complete physiology. As you find your energy levels rising you are going to want to do more exercise.

Once you have eliminated non-food completely you are going to feel positive about what you eat. That positive effect will show in your wellbeing. The thing that is going to intrigue you most is how you ever managed to survive at all on - poisonous fat, sugar and salt that you once regarded as *food.* Non-food has to become a thing of the past.

Having eliminated the negative we are now in an advantageous position to accentuate the positive.

" They say time changes things,
but you actually have to change them yourself." - Andy Warhol

57

Human Proportions

To achieve human proportions we do not need to train like Olympic athletes or live on a Spartan diet. We need to exercise for twenty to thirty minutes a day and eat real-food in human proportions.

Fortunately we were given the ultimate guide to measuring food in human proportions - our hands – which are in direct proportion to our bodies.

If you hold your hands together in front of you, the amount of real-food you can hold in both hands constitutes a meal. It's simple!

We need to eat four meals a day, at four-hour intervals, whenever possible, to maintain our metabolism at its optimum level.

The first thought that jumps into the mind of anyone who has ever attempted dieting before is - what if I'm hungry between meals?

The simple answer is, if you have been yo-yo dieting you might initially need to eat extra fruit and vegetables between meals, but the operative word is 'might' as it will probably have more to do with an imagined or emotional need than actual hunger.

We understandably all have an underlying primal fear of being hungry, as with all underlying fears they are easier to overcome once they are recognised. Primal fears are an essential part of our being.

The questions we must ask ourselves are: Am I hungry?

Do I just think I'm hungry? Or, is it that, I'm actually thirsty?

There is no greater arrogance than to attempt to assess the depth of emotion that any individual feels. You are the only person capable of knowing the depth of your own feelings. But you are in more of a position to clarify, how you actually feel, when you know that outside influences such as alcohol, non-food and junk food are not clouding your judgement. Once you are eating only real food, in human proportions, you will begin to realise, quite quickly, that any food addiction you might have had is disappearing.

The key measurement to eating in human proportions is that a meal consists of what your two hands can hold. The key measurement in overcoming emotional eating, is to live - *'One day at a time!'*

" Inch by Inch is a cinch – yard by yard is hard." - American Proverb.

Breakfast is the most important meal of the day; it kicks our metabolism into action and powers up our brain. Breakfast has to be a substantial meal, as it needs to fuel our system from four to six hours.

Firstly we look at the basis of a breakfast that you should not tire of, and because its amazing benefits should be eaten four to five mornings a week. The main constituent of this breakfast is:

- Oats -

Oats are easily digested, they contain zinc and potassium, an essential nerve conductor, also magnesium a protein synthesiser involved in energy production. Oats contain the amino acid cysteine, which removes heavy metals from the body. The protein content of oats is high, thirteen percent. The silica in oats aids healing and most importantly oats actually lower LDL cholesterol. A soluble fibre they bind with bile acids that are made from cholesterol; these cholesterol laden, bile acids are then excreted. Further cholesterol is then wrested from the blood to make more bile acids and the whole process is then replicated clearing the blood of life threatening LDL cholesterol. Soluble fibre helps regulate blood sugar, which levels out energy and provides stamina. Oats are excellent food for cancer patients undergoing chemotherapy.

If the giant pharmaceutical companies had the monopoly on oats their status would change from a food to a medicine and you would be looking at paying many times the price for this traditionally inexpensive food which grows abundantly even on the poorest soil.

When you buy a packet of oats, always buy organic, what you buy is what you get, one hundred percent pure organic oats with no added ingredients. To ensure that there is no depletion of the B and E vitamin content, oats are best eaten raw. Just allow them to soak for five to ten minutes in cold water and they are ready to eat.

Perspective and balance are important, as you could have too much of a good thing, not because of their calorific value which is minimal for such a satisfying food, but because of their content of phytic acid which taken in excess will stop the absorption of iron, calcium and zinc from other foods. (Oats can be soaked overnight.)

We will be adding a couple of tablespoons of wheat germ to the oats.

- Wheat Germ -

When people talk about the goodness being taken out of white bread, wheat germ is that goodness, the most nutritious part of the wheat. It takes the production of thirty-six pounds of white flour to produce one pound of wheat germ.

Amazingly, humans eat white bread and thoroughbred racehorses are fed on wheat germ. Wheat germ is one of the best sources of vitamin E – which the body can only store for a short time. Vitamin E retards cellular ageing due to oxidation and, enhances oxygen supply to the body, increasing stamina and eliminating fatigue. As an anticoagulant it dissolves blood clots. It is a natural diuretic and decreases high blood pressure. It is hardly surprising that thoroughbred racehorses look so good!

The reason food producers remove the wheat germ from wheat is shelf life. In the majority of cases, the shorter the shelf life of a food, the more nutritious it is. Wheat germ is the life force of wheat.

Use the lunacy of the situation in your favour – buy the wheat germ and leave the depleted, artificially enhanced white bread where it belongs on the shelf.

Wheat germ is high in phytic acid, which inhibits the absorption of iron, calcium and zinc. To counteract this, ensure that you counterbalance your intake of wheat germ with foods high in Vitamin C.

Once opened, keep wheat germ refrigerated, many people who have wheat intolerance are not affected by wheat germ.

Oats and wheat germ are the basis of breakfast four to five times a week, there could be nothing easier to prepare, all you have to add is as much fresh fruit as you like.

This breakfast is going to help you start your day with a constant supply of energy, while filling you with the most nutritious food on the planet. In the league of good food this is as good as it gets!

We now take the opportunity to look at exactly why we are recommended to eat five pieces of fruit a day. On this diet we will try to exceed that amount, and the reasons are about to make themselves very obvious.

- Apples -

I'm not sure if the apple was mentioned in the Bible before the fig leaf, but either way they have been around for a long time, make sure that you eat at least two apples a day. The antioxidant effect of the flavonoid querectin, found mainly in the apple's skin, is excellent for the treatment of gout and joint problems. Richer than any other fruit in Vitamin E they help prevent the oxidation of fat compounds. The chlorogenic acid content is thought to help fight the formation of cancer cells. Low in the glycaemic index they are excellent for diabetics. If you want to snack between meals, go ahead. The pectin in apples is one of the greatest aids to digestion. Querectin is an exceptional antioxidant, which lowers the risk of heart attacks and strokes. In a study conducted in Finland regular apple eaters, had over a fifty-five percent less chance of having a stroke.

- Apricots -

Originating in China, apricots were introduced to the wider world by Alexander the Great. Dried apricots, received almost legendary status at the hands of the Hunzakuts who live in the Hunza Valley in North Pakistan. Apricots form part of the Hunza's Spartan diet. Aided by the fact that they have no birth certificates, their remarkable longevity is *slightly* exaggerated. Regardless, they are a remarkably healthy race and even after the exaggeration factor is reduced by forty years they still live well into their nineties. Apricots contain iron and fibre and are a fine source of potassium. Potassium helps prevent and relieve high blood pressure, and cannot be stored in the body, we need a regular supply. Severe potassium deficiency leads to mental confusion, heart attacks and strokes. Apricots are a wonderful source of the carotenoid, beta-carotene, which enhances eyesight.
Because of their concentrated energy, food and medicinal value, dried apricots were part of the American astronauts diet on some space flights. Dried or fresh apricots are part of our extensive armoury against disease.

To get the maximum nutritional value from dried fruits eat them regularly in small amounts and ensure that you always eat them in conjunction with fresh fruit to extract the most from their nutritional value. Always wash dried fruit, as it removes excess sugar that forms on them and any alfatoxins.

- Bananas -

Half a billion people in Africa and Asia depend on bananas as their staple food. Bananas are an excellent source of potassium, which constitutes five percent of the mineral content of the body. Potassium helps maintain healthy blood pressure and heart function. Bananas contain the alkaloid compound bufotenine that helps stimulate the production of serotonin, which enhances mood. An indicator of how easily digested bananas are, is that they are one of the first solid foods fed to babies. When your strength is flagging, do what professional sportsman do, eat a banana, it provides a steady flow of energy.

- Blueberries -

These deep purple berries have the highest antioxidant capacity of all fresh fruit and are an excellent anti-bacterial because of the amount of anthocyanin they contain, anthocyanin produces blue and violet colours in fruit and plants. Blueberries, a natural anti-bacterium also provide a source of natural aspirin. For centuries they have been a remedy for stomach complaints, and in the treatment of diarrhoea and urinary infections such as cystitis. The flavonoids in blueberries strengthen blood capillaries and aid circulation.

When looking at the pros and cons of flying produce around the world blueberries, because of their medicinal properties, justify their journey. Had Ponce de Leon managed to find the fountain of youth, you can be sure the water would have been deep purple.

Blueberries are available in your supermarket all the year round, take advantage of this and eat them two or three times a week, their benefits are outstanding. .

- Cranberries -

Cranberries have many of the same qualities as blueberries and are used as a recognised treatment for urinary infections. They are a powerful antioxidant.

Antioxidants are the body's front line troops in fighting free radicals. Free radicals cause damage to your cells leading to diseases like cancer. That is why we need to eat fruit and vegetables daily!

Cranberries contain the flavonoids querectin and myricetin the very dark varieties contain a third flavonoid kaempferol; all three help stop damage to the lining of blood vessels.

In most instances it is far better to eat fresh fruit, than it is to drink fruit juice. You always want the complete fruit, as fresh as possible, containing all of the fruit's enzymes. Cranberries are an exception to this rule.

Cranberries have to be cooked to release their juice. Always look for 'pure cranberry juice.' You do not want to buy any juice that is labelled as a 'juice drink' as this means the juice has been adulterated. When buying any kind of fruit juice, the label must read 'pure juice.' Cranberries are not just for Christmas - they are for life!

- Dates -

Niacin, one of the B vitamins, is one of the main constituents of dates; a deficiency of niacin is responsible for the disease pellagra, whose symptoms include weakness, depression, dermatitis and diarrhoea. On the downside dates trigger migraines in some people.

- Figs -

The Romans thought so highly of figs that they outlawed their export. Fresh figs perish easily, usually a sign of abundant goodness in a fruit. Over ninety percent of the world's productions of figs are dried. Dried figs are high in calcium. A glass of milk contains 116mg of calcium – four dried figs contain the same amount. Figs are also rich in, potassium, magnesium and iron. Japanese researchers have isolated anti cancer agent benzaldehyde from figs, which helps shrink tumors.

- Grapefruit -

The grapefruit diet was one of the earliest fad diets, it first appeared in the 1930's, known as the Hollywood diet, and it keeps getting resurrected. There's no magic enzyme in grapefruits, but they are a fabulous fruit, and they definitely need to be part of your diet for all the right reasons. The finest grapefruits are the red-fleshed varieties that come from Trinidad and Florida. They contain cholesterol-lowering pectin and they are also excellent sources of limonoids and naringin, which have cancer-fighting properties. Grapefruits also inhibit the formation of kidney stones. If you are taking any prescription drugs check with your doctor that it is alright to eat grapefruit, as they can have an effect on drug absorption.

- Guavas -

Guavas are not always available in the United Kingdom but they have to be mentioned because of their high content of lycopene which is one of the strongest anti-oxidants. Israeli scientists have found in laboratory studies that lycopene blocks the growth of lung and breast cancer cells. In a major study into prostate cancer at Harvard it was found that men with increased lycopene in their diets reduced the risk of prostate cancer by over forty percent. (An excellent, always available, source of lycopene is tomatoes, but they have to be cooked to release their lycopene) Guavas also have an exceptional amount of dietary fibre.

- Grapes -

Grapes contain ellagic acid, a phytochemical that destroys hydrocarbons, the cancer causing chemicals in cigarettes. Red and black varieties are best as their skins contain resveratrol, which inhibits the formation of blood clots. They also contain the anti oxidant quercetin. As with all fruit, wash grapes well before eating.

- Honey -

You can be sure that primitive man would have been enthralled by honey, and utilised it to the best of his ability. Two thousand years ago, the Romans used honey as an antibiotic. Local honey is often used as a first resort in treating hay fever.

There are thousands of different types of honey and their subtle differences and healing properties are just being realised by modern medicine.

The native New Zealanders, the Maoris, use manuka honey as a treatment for ulcers, boils, cuts and grazes. Scientists have recently discovered that manuka honey kills the helicobacter pylori bug, and is a better cure for gastric ulcers than drug based medicine. As a food it should be used in moderation, but often.

- Kiwi Fruit -

Chinese Gooseberries, Yang Tao, Kiwi fruit are an exceptional source of vitamin C and can be stored for months with very little depletion of their vitamin content. In addition they are a source of lutein, which helps prevent cataracts and macular degeneration. Kiwi fruit are high in copper, vital for infant growth and brain development. Kiwis contain more potassium than bananas - they also contain vitamin E and magnesium. Kiwi fruit should be eaten daily, take full advantage of the highly concentrated nutrients in this amazing fruit.

Kiwi fruit are available all the year round. If, in the future, a licence should ever be needed, to justify that a fruit is nutritionally worthy enough to travel, the kiwi will have no trouble in attaining a licence. Dr. Paul Lachance of Rutgers University, New Brunswick, N.J., established that ounce for ounce; the kiwi fruit was the most nutritionally dense of the twenty-seven most commonly consumed fruits. (The kiwi was closely followed by papaya and mango.) (The avocado would seem to have been left out of this list of commonly consumed fruits, as it might have been assumed to be a vegetable, a common enough mistake to make, the avocados' considerable attributes including its amazing nutrient density are extolled later in this book.)

- Lemons & Limes -

British sailors gained the nickname 'Limeys' in the 18th century, when Scottish naval surgeon, James Lind discovered that eating citrus fruit cured scurvy. Prior to this the disease had ravaged mariners since man first went to sea. Citrus fruit is full of vitamin C, which helps the body manufacture collagen the material that bonds cells together in order to heal cuts and wounds.

Lemons and limes are indispensable when added to food as their unique flavour lessens the need for salt.

The peel of lemons and limes contain limonene, which increases enzyme production in the liver that helps remove cancer-causing chemicals from the body. Before trying to remove the zest from lemon or lime peel, ensure you wash them carefully in hot water to remove any wax and preservatives which growers use to ensure their shelf life.

- Melons -

It could well be that the complete human race owes its existence to melons. There is very little rainfall in the Kalahari Desert and our distant ancestors, the San Bushmen (see page 49) survived by eating Tsama Melons that grow just under the surface of the ground. Tsama melons were the Bushmen's main source of water, prized more than the diamonds that littered the surface of the parched earth that was their home.

Melons are a wonderful source of potassium, which lowers blood pressure. The correlation goes something like this. The more potassium you eat the more sodium you lose and the lower your blood pressure is likely to be. It is essential to eat potassium rich foods regularly to allow your body to balance your salt intake. Potassium and sodium facilitate the transmission of nerve impulses.

The Chinese have used melon as an anticoagulant for thousands of years, so it comes as no surprise that melons work wonders for the cardiovascular system.

- Peaches and Nectarines -

When asked what was the finest thing he'd ever encountered, in two thousand years, Mcl Brooks' and Carl Reiners' enigmatic creation, the Two Thousand Year Old Man replied, 'Nectarines!'

Sometimes mistakenly thought of as a recent hybrid between a peach and plum, nectarines have actually been about for over two thousand years. Peaches and Nectarines are luscious and easy to digest, everything of a sensual experience they are rich in beta-carotene and vitamin C.

- Cherries -

Before fruit took to refrigerated-flight and became available all year round, cherries used to evoke the feeling of summer, this was before the polythene bag replaced the brown paper bag and life seemed simpler, in effect when life was, 'just a bowl of cherries!'

Cherries contain a compound called perillyl alcohol, which was found to be one of the best cures for mammary cancer in laboratory animals in tests carried out in The University of Wisconsin's Medical School.

Cherries also contain, querectin and vitamins A, E and C. Eating cherries 8oz of cherries per day lowers uric acid so they are excellent in the treatment of gout, which has been making a comeback with people on high protein, meat diets.

- Kumquats -

Kumquats are high in potassium, calcium and vitamins A and C. Resembling a miniature orange they can be eaten entirely, their delicate skin is sweet and their fruit is tart. Cut these miniature fruits in half and smear them with honey, place them under the grill for less than a minute and you have the Chinese remedy for colds and flu.

To maximise their absorption, nuts are best eaten with fruits rich in vitamin C. Nuts are an integral part of our diet, we need to eat them little and often. Nuts contain more vitamin E than any other food. They also contain copper and magnesium. Nuts are high in good fats - monounsaturated and polyunsaturated.

Coconuts contain Lauric acid, which raises the metabolism, put this evidence together with the evidence earlier in the book for almonds and peanuts and we begin to realise that fixed calorific values, and the actual energy these ostensible values produce in a human being, are far from exact. In a nutshell calorific values are not what they are cracked up to be!

The nutritional value of nuts is colossal, nutritional density exceeds itself when it comes to nuts; that is why they have to be fundamental to our diet.

Many years ago, Edgar Cayce said that eating five almonds a day would ward off cancer. Modern medical evidence is beginning to prove him right, in a report from the American Institute for Cancer Research and the World Cancer Research Fund it was stated that: 'Diets high in nuts could prove to be protective against some cancers.' Paul Davis, PhD, lead researcher in the study said: "Not only did whole almonds inhibit colon cancer precursor cells from developing, but we were gratified to see that they were significantly more effective than wheat bran, widely believed to be protective against this type of cancer."

In a report in the British Medical Journal, Harvard School of Public Health researchers found that women who ate more than five ounces of nuts a day, had a thirty two percent *lower* risk of having a heart attack compared to women who avoided nuts completely. Balance this evidence against the increased risk of a heart attack from eating meat, and it is obvious where our supply of protein needs to come from.

- Almonds -

Almonds are rich in protein and calcium; there are high levels of antioxidants in almond skins that are initially released when we chew them. When we chew almonds thoroughly we begin to combine the polyphenols in the almonds skin with the vitamin E content of the almond, producing a powerful combatant against heart disease and cancer. Therefore, avoid blanched almonds, as they do not have the healing potential of almonds in their original state.

- Brazil Nuts -

Brazil nuts have about two thousand times the selenium content of any other nut. The trace element selenium is a powerful antioxidant that discourages the ageing process and stimulates the immune system. Brazil nuts are one of the most nutritionally dense foods on the planet, they have a high zinc content and also contain magnesium, phosphorous, copper and iron.

Brazil nuts need to be well chewed, and eaten often and sparingly, you have to regard nuts as a medicine in their own right, eaten in the small amounts, regularly, they will prove the theory that in many instances less is definitely more!

- Cashews -

The Cashew tree originated in Brazil and is related to the pistachio and the mango. Cashews are rich in iron and zinc; improved iron levels lead to better concentration. Improved zinc levels lead to a better sex life. As tempting as it might be, do not add salt to nuts, we need to eat small amounts of nuts regularly, adding salt makes you want to eat far too many nuts at one time, which is definitely not our objective. We are eating nuts as a preventative medicine, not as a palliative.

- Chestnuts -

The Romans made flour out of chestnuts. Apicius the only surviving classical cookbook surviving from the time of the Roman Empire describes a dish made from chestnuts and lentils. Chestnuts have the lowest fat content of any nut, and are an excellent base, for making nourishing nut-roasts.

- Macadamia Nuts -

Macadamia nuts are rich in manganese, essential for sex hormone formation. Manganese is important as it helps form thyroxine, the principal hormone of the thyroid gland that stimulates metabolism and is essential for growth and development. Macadamia nuts also contain palmitoleic acid, which aids in fat metabolism.

- Walnuts -

Walnuts have to be part of our daily diet! According to a study by the University of Oslo, walnuts are cited as the largest single source of antioxidants next to rosehips, which contain the most.

The Unites States Food and Drug Administration support the health claim that walnuts may reduce the risk of heart disease. Walnuts are high in Omega 3 oil. Walnuts also contain ellagic acid, a cancer fighting anti oxidant; they are also a good source of copper, which helps make melanin the skin pigment. Pecans are second cousins to walnuts and share many of their qualities.

Nuts are an important adjunct to your diet, at the risk of being repetitive: For the best effect eat them often and sparingly!

Some nut allergies are dangerous, but fortunately they are rare.

Women who are pregnant should consult their doctor before making any radical change in their diet, as overindulgence in any one particular food is not advised.

- Pistachio Nuts -

Pistachios enhance your sex life, as they contain valuable amounts of zinc. Zinc is essential to the immune system; they also contain potassium, vitamin E, calcium and Iron.

- Peanuts -

Peanuts are legumes; strictly speaking they are closer to a pea than a nut. Protein rich peanut butter has exceptional health benefits. Served on multigrain, wholemeal bread or toast, the full potential of its protein value is released.

In a study conducted recently at the Pennsylvania State University a peanut rich, unsaturated fat diet resulted in favourable heart benefits. Reducing cardiovascular disease by fourteen percent.

In a previous study at Harvard School of Public Health and Brigham and Women's Hospital in Boston they found that three times as many people were able to stick to a healthy moderate fat weight loss diet than those following low fat weight loss diets.

Both the above diets had peanut butter as their main constituent, as opposed to butter or margarine.

Apart from raising your metabolism, peanuts have a high satiety value and leave you feeling full and contented. Peanuts are also very low on the glycaemic index and ideal for diabetics, giving a slow and constant release of energy.

Peanuts are an exceptional source of resveratrol. Animal studies have shown that resveratrol can inhibit the growth of the damaged cells, which cause cancer.

The protein power in peanuts is on a par with meat, without any of the hazardous side effects.

- Rosehips -

Rosehips are an exceptional source of vitamin C and antioxidants. They are a renowned treatment for headaches and mouth ulcers. Flu sufferers should drink rosehip tea, as it is excellent in relieving the unpleasant symptoms of an infected respiratory tract.

- Oranges -

Oranges would only need recommendation to somebody from another planet. Nature performed a brilliant advertising job when it packaged the orange; you only have to see a ripe orange to want to reach out and grab it! Along with Clementines, Mineaolas, Satsumas, Tangerines, Tangelos, Ortaniques and Ugli-Fruit. These fruits are packed with vitamin C and betacarotene.

The Orange takes fourth place in the list of nutritionally dense fruits. Oranges help improve iron absorption and are one of the foremost cancer inhibitors, containing: carotenoids, flavonoids and terpenes.

Eating the complete fruit, is far better than buying fruit juice, as the pulp of the fruit contains pectin which lowers cholesterol and protects your arteries. The body does not store vitamin C so we need to replenish this important vitamin daily.

- Papayas -

Papayas were a close second behind the kiwi fruit in the list of nutritional density. In the tropics they heal wounds by placing the inner side of papaya skin directly to the wound. Papayas contain papain, which promotes the breakdown of protein and is instrumental in alleviating digestive disorders and detoxification. Papain is excellent for your teeth as it helps to loosen bacteria that bonds to tooth enamel, making it easier to brush bacteria away. Papayas have a very high content of vitamin C.

- Passion Fruit -

Passion Fruits are also known as Granadillas, meaning little pomegranate in Spanish. Passion fruit are excellent for the nervous system, relieving insomnia and depression. They are high in potassium, vitamin A and Iron.

- Persimmons -

Persimmons, Kaki, Lampshi, are the national fruit of Japan. Although they are known as 'apples of the orient' they have more of the feel of a tomato about them. They can only be eaten when they are fully ripe; when fully ripe they become almost translucent. When they are ready to eat, cut off the top with a knife and scoop them out with a teaspoon.

The Chinese believe that Persimmons aid longevity. This could well be true as they are an exceptional source of vitamin A, which builds resistance to respiratory infections and shortens the duration of disease.

- Pineapple -

Pineapples have a high content of manganese, essential in the making of collagen, which helps form connective tissue. People deficient in manganese develop bone problems. The enzyme bromelain in pineapple aids digestion as it breaks down protein. It is important to eat fresh pineapple as bromelain depletes in the juicing and canning process. Bromelain is a powerful anti-inflammatory and has a positive effect on anyone suffering from arthritis.

- Pomegranates -

Once they are ripe, there is really only one way to eat a pomegranate, that is to keep rolling and applying pressure to the fruit in your hands, until the contents are pulped, then make a small incision at the bottom of the fruit and suck out the juice, once the juice is removed, open the fruit and do your best to eat the seeds and pulp. How any child could prefer a man made confection than this wonderfully messy fruit is beyond understanding. Pomegranates are a potent source of ellagic acid, a cancer fighting antioxidant; they are also full of vitamin C.

- Pears -

Pears contain lignin, an insoluble fibre that extracts cholesterol from your body. Lignin effectively traps cholesterol molecules in the intestine, before they become absorbed in the bloodstream. They also contain the mineral boron that helps to strengthen bones. Boron is also a brain food; research has show that in tests boron increased both memory and attention span. There are traces of boron in most fruits and by eating your quota of a variety of fruits each day your brain can work at its optimum level. The antibacterial acids in pears have successfully inhibited the growth of the Shigella-sonnei bacteria, which causes severe gastroenteritis.

- Plums and Prunes -

Plums and dried prunes are a potent source of ferulic acid; they also contain phenolic phytochemicals, making them an important antioxidant. Plums and prunes offer a high level of defence against free radicals. Plums and prunes are also high in iron and potassium. Prunes contain a natural sugar called sorbitol, which like fibre soaks up water, this together with dihidroxyphenylisatin, stimulates the intestines, causing them to contract, ensuring regular bowel movements.

Dried prunes have double the substantial antioxidant value of fresh blueberries.

- Pumpkin Seeds -

Pumpkin seeds are rich in zinc, potassium, omega 3 oils, and iron. They go rancid quite quickly; once you have bought them keep them in an airtight container and use as soon as possible. They contain as much protein as meat.

As with all foods rich in zinc they have a positive effect on the immune system and fertility.

- Raspberries -

The Romans used raspberries as a cure for tonsillitis, and they haven't lost any of their potency. Australian Scientist, Dr. Heather Cavanagh at Charles Sturt University, New South Wales, Australia, has verified that Raspberry Juice can kill the bacteria that causes gastroenteritis. They are a powerful antioxidant that protects against heart disease and cancer. Raspberries also contain natural aspirin. With a much more defined taste loganberries parallel the qualities of the raspberry, and are a hybrid of the blackberry and raspberry. Raspberries are closely related to strawberries.

- Strawberries -

Strawberries, as with all fresh berries, need to be eaten as quickly as possible to gain their full nutrient value; squeezing a little lemon on them brings out their flavour. An excellent source of salicylates, natural aspirin, they are a medicine in their own right. Strawberries are extremely high in vitamin C and pectin. Some sufferers of rheumatoid arthritis have claimed that they relieve their symptoms.

- Tomatoes - -

In the Galapagos Islands, Darwin's favourite haunt, tomatoes that are as black as blackberries grow wild. There are hundreds of varieties of tomatoes, they are universally popular and one of the easiest crops to grow, they are an integral part of the Mediterranean diet.

Tomatoes need to find their way into our diet every day. They contain lycopene, which is released when they are cooked. Along with olive oil, tomatoes are one of the major ingredients that make the Mediterranean diet so successful. Research has proved that people with high levels of lycopene in their blood have a much lower risk of contracting most forms of cancer. Tomato puree, canned tomatoes and all forms of non-adulterated tomato sauces are fine, as lycopene is released when tomatoes are cooked. The beneficial effects of this fruit, usually regarded as a vegetable, are immense and cannot be overstated.

When the Conquistadors appropriated the Incas' gold they also discovered the Avocado pear. To describe the avocado as a super-nutrient is an understatement. To say that an avocado is calorific, without taking into account its amazing nutritional density, does an injustice to the avocado and to anyone who might be persuaded to deny themselves one of the most valuable nutrient rich foods on the planet.

Fortunately, our interest in calories is only academic, as we are only interested in nutritional density and the health giving benefits of food, but from a purely academic point of view, cheese is 40% saturated fat which creates bad cholesterol, Avocado is 25% monounsaturated fat which lowers bad cholesterol.

The satiety value of the avocado is unparalleled it fulfils your craving for fat and ensures you have no interest in non-foods and that fulfilment is sustained. The avocado is 25% protein, the highest protein content of any fruit. Avocados are rich in vitamin C, vitamin E, Vitamin B6 and riboflavin.

The avocado contains glutathione, a powerful antioxidant shown to block over thirty different carcinogens - the avocado fights cancer.

The avocado, in measured amounts, is excellent for diabetics as it contains a type of natural sugar called mannoheptulose, which lowers insulin levels as opposed to raising them the way ordinary sugar does.

Simple to prepare, you just mash them with a little salt and pepper to taste. The Japanese mash them with grated horseradish.

In West Africa and South America the avocado is used as baby food, it contains all the essential amino acids to be a complete food.

The media should take great care before talking vacuously about calorific values, without taking nutritional values into account, as their input can do immeasurable damage to vulnerable young people, struggling with an abstract concept, which can all too often turn into an obsessive eating disorder.

" You have the situation where girls of eight want to diet,
at twelve they can tell you the fat content of an avocado
but they don't know what constitutes a healthy meal. "
- Mary Evans Young.

- Breakfast -

There is no substitute for knowledge. Knowing the nutritional goodness of our food has an amazing psychological effect on us.

Knowing that our breakfast is abundant with antioxidants and vitamins makes a total difference to our outlook. We are administering preventative medicine to ourselves and building up our immune systems. We are in command of our lives, while eating fulfilling, nourishing food that leaves us satisfied.

We are also eating in human proportions, knowing that the meal we have just eaten will carry us through to our next meal, in four to six hours time. There is no guilt attached to our diet, we are doing the very best we can, it's simple but it works.

Breakfast fires up your metabolism and powers your brain. We have the most amazing choice of fruit and nuts to add to the basic oatmeal and wheat germ base. Go sparingly with the nuts, but make sure that you have some each and every day.

You might want to add pumpkin seeds or linseeds to your breakfast, or to make a change you could easily add some dried fruit, soaked over night, (when you are soaking dried fruit overnight try adding fresh lemon or lime juice for flavour.)

To reiterate, the base for breakfast is a bowl of organic oats soaked for five or ten minutes in cold water, with two tablespoons of wheat germ added. With as wide a variety of fruit as possible and a few mixed nuts.

- Linseeds -

Linseeds come from the flax plant and are the highest known source of Omega 3 fatty acids derived from a plant. Linseeds ease menopausal symptoms and are excellent for the digestive system. Linseeds are best kept in the refrigerator for freshness.

Alternative Breakfasts

On the days you decide not to eat the mainstay breakfast of oats, wheat germ, fruit and nuts there are many alternatives.

Multi seed, wholemeal bread or rye bread, is fine, when we talk about human proportions in bread, we are talking about a couple of slices, plain or toasted per day. Spread with peanut butter and honey, and eaten with a banana or any other fruits that you might fancy.

A couple of slices of toast with grilled tomatoes and mushrooms, plus any fruit to follow is another alternative.

Baked beans are excellent; it's just the sauce that's a problem as the sauce is filled with sugar, salt and additives. There is a way around the problem, if you can't find baked beans in your supermarket that are additive free, just buy the economy kind; the beans don't know that they are travelling economy class, place them in a sieve and wash off the offending sauce with cold water. Open a can of chopped tomatoes that are additive free, pour away the excess fluid and add the tomatoes to your beans and cook them; the tomatoes ensure you get your lycopene. This way you can have beans on toast without all of the unnecessary sugar and additives. Haricot beans are available without sauce but, because of relative less demand, they are more expensive.

If you are partial to a pair of kippers, they are an excellent source of omega 3. Although they are high in sodium, we definitely need some salt, this way we get our quota of salt with a nutritional bonus.

Bubble and squeak, makes a fulfilling breakfast, using up yesterdays mashed potatoes, and vegetables, mix them together with some olive oil to bind them into rissole proportions and lightly fry them in olive oil. Served with grilled tomatoes, it's a nutritious breakfast that will tempt children when other breakfasts are declined.

A bowl of hot porridge made simply with boiling water and a little honey added, is an unbeatable winter breakfast.

- Soup -

If there's any food that soothes the soul as much as homemade soup, it has unfortunately evaded me. Before we go through the nutrients in vegetables, we look at one of the mainstays of our diet, thick vegetable soup.

To make creamy soup you don't need dairy food, just a few potatoes blended with a little olive oil, they make soup creamy. All you need is a saucepan and an electric blender.

Because of the variety of vegetables and herbs available you cannot possibly grow tired of soup as a meal. Any one vegetable can be predominant, any mixture melds together, the possibilities are endless, the nutritional value astounding.

You cannot make too much, as it tastes better the next day. If you think that sticking to a diet of real-food will be difficult when working away from home, think again! A thermos flask full of hot vegetable soup is the most fulfilling meal you could possibly have.

Peel three or four medium potatoes and cut into small pieces, chop up an onion and a few cloves of garlic, chop up a generous handful of fresh parsley. Alternate the fresh herbs when making different soups, basil, sage, thyme, and coriander. Add olive oil.

Let your intuition guide you through the soup making process, it is much like painting on canvas, all you need, are the basic elements and you create the work of art. No vegetable is exempt from this soup, chose whatever you like, just chop them up and throw them in. Bring to the boil and simmer for ten minutes. Place them in the blender and blitz them, then pour them back into the saucepan, add a tablespoon of Miso (Miso is a fermented Soya-bean paste of Japanese origin, rich in digestive enzymes and high in protein.) Cook gently for a further five minutes and the soup is completed. The predominant vegetable decides the flavour: Tomato and Basil, Carrot and Coriander, Leek and Potato, Broccoli, Beetroot and Onion, Shitake mushroom soup, (Use fresh and dried mushrooms, also add other varieties of mushroom)

" *Soup is a lot like a family, each ingredient enhances the others, each has its own characteristics, and it needs to simmer to reach full flavour.*"
- Marge Kennedy

We are primarily interested in fish that are low in the food chain, as they are far less likely to be contaminated by dioxins and mercury. In basic terms, to generate each pound in weight a large fish needs to consume ten pounds of small fish. Then take into account that large fish have a longer life span than small fish, which gives them a greater opportunity to get contaminated. Therefore, large fish contain more than ten times the mercury of small fish populating the same seas. Marlin, tuna, swordfish and shark are not on our agenda because of their greater likelihood of being contaminated.

We are not interested in farmed fish, as they have no seabed to feed on, only toxic waste. The man-made system in which they exist is far inferior to a natural ecological system. Some farmed fish are fed on synthetic canthaxanthin to enhance their colour; this chemical is being placed into the food chain merely for appearance. If there were any attempt to use it as a direct additive to food, it would be banned.

We must not allow the fact that some fish are polluted to stop us eating unpolluted fish, a food that is essential to our wellbeing.

Fresh and smoked salmon from the pacific are fine. Most U.K tinned salmon, originates from the Pacific and is of excellent quality.

The fish we are mainly interested in are, mackerel, herring, sardines, trout and salmon; both tinned and fresh. These are a prime source of Omega 3 oils and are extremely important to our health.

A tin of sardines, is an unbelievable power pack of nutritional goodness, they contain over four hundred milligrams of high quality calcium plus protein, iron, zinc and omega 3. Always buy them in olive oil as it adds omega 6 and, if you buy them in virgin olive oil, it adds omega 9.

Omega 3, with either omega 6, or 9, compliment each other and will improve many aspects of your health. Within a few weeks you will notice that small cuts heal faster, your skin tone and hair will improve and your pain threshold will increase.

The U.K. supply of white fish such as cod, haddock, sole or plaice come mainly from the North Atlantic, they are an excellent source of complete protein, and should be eaten grilled or steamed at least once or twice a week. Shellfish are fine if not farmed.

Beans have outstanding food values: Fresh, canned, dried, or sprouting, they have to be wholehcartedly incorporated into your diet.

Nutritionally, fibre rich and low in fat, beans are at the forefront of fighting cancer as they contain: Lignans, saponins, phytic acid, protease inhibitors plus isoflavones, genistein and daidzein.

We begin with soya beans an excellent source of protein; in fact records show that they have been the main source of protein in China for over four thousand years. Pound for pound soya beans contain twice the protein of meat and ten times the protein of milk. This vegetable protein is far easier to assimilate than animal protein.

In the Second World War, when there were meat shortages in the United States, they doubled their soya bean production. Evidence indicates that soya beans were one of the first cultivated crops grown by man. They contain omega 3 oils.

The nutritional power that can be released from beans is profound. The Chinese have sprouted Soya beans for four thousand years. Four thousand years before junk food was invented!

It is quite simple to sprout beans and very much worth the effort, as you could not possibly eat fresher vegetables than those that are actually growing. Always sprout a mixed variety at the same time, including, mung beans, soya beans and chickpeas. Add any other sprouting beans and grains for a variety of wonderful flavours.

If you are looking for the vegetable at the top of the super nutrient list, sprouting beans will always get the vote as they contain: Vitamins A, C, D, E, K and B complex, plus - iron, calcium, manganese, potassium and phosphorous. When you sprout beans you multiply their nutrient value immensely. Vitamin C increases over five hundred per cent during sprouting, their nutrient density actually increases while they are in your refrigerator.

You can buy a bean sprouting kit at any good health food shop. This means you have the basis of a fresh salad on hand all the time with a depth of nutritional density that is astounding.

Sprouting beans should be eaten with as many meals as possible, there is only one-way to describe them, they are 'The life force'!

- Beans, Legumes/Pulses and Grains -

Beans are an excellent source of protein when eaten with rice, brown basmati rice is excellent, as it is low on the glycaemic index and gives an even flow of energy, making beans and brown rice an excellent base for a meal, when cooking for a diabetic.

There are endless varieties of beans, aduki beans, haricot beans, navy beans, butter beans, mung beans, black eye beans, broad beans, canellini beans, fava beans, flagelot beans, borlotti beans, pinto beans and red kidney beans just to mention a few. Try them all, as there will be subtle differences in their nutritional value and you want as much variety in your diet as possible. Beans are high in soluble fibre, which reduces bad cholesterol.

Chickpeas are the main ingredient of hummus; eaten with wholemeal pita bread they are a fine source of protein. Chickpeas can also be sprouted releasing more health giving enzymes.

Peas are the richest source of B1, surpassing liver, which aficionados of meat regard as a *wonder nutrient.* Peas also have a very high zinc content, accompanied by brown basmati rice an excellent nutritional balance is created. Once again ideal food for diabetics, as a rule, food that is good for diabetics is excellent for everyone, as it gives sustained energy over a prolonged period. Frozen peas do not lose any of their nutrients. Blended with potatoes, olive oil and garlic, peas make a wonderful health giving soup.

Lentils are a good source of protein and Iron and contain isoflavones. Asian women suffer less menopausal symptoms than women in the west, as they eat foods rich in isoflavones; once again mix lentils with brown rice to enhance nutrient values. Combining the right foods ensures that you get all the protein that you need. Lentils are extremely versatile and can be used in casseroles and soups.

Quinoa originated in the Andes, it contains more protein than meat and more usable calcium than milk and has an ideal balance of amino acids. Quinoa flakes are excellent added to soups; bought in grain form, Quinoa can be sprouted, which multiplies its enzyme value.

Sprouted Quinoa contains, Vitamins A, B6, B12, C, D, E and K, biotin, folic acid, niacin, pantothenic acid, selenium and zinc, chromium, copper and magnesium; it's a nutritional powerhouse.

- Artichokes -

Artichokes are excellent for anyone suffering with liver or gall bladder problems as they contain cynarin, which lowers blood cholesterol and improves the digestion process. They also contain the powerful antioxidant silymarin, which blocks the effect of cancer causing free radicals. Silymarin extract is used to fight liver disease. Artichokes are also a fine source of magnesium, which is essential for healthy heart function. Pregnant women, who need to ensure that they eat enough folate-rich foods, should add artichokes to their diet. Frozen artichoke hearts retain their folate.

To the uninitiated globe artichokes might seem like something of a struggle to eat, they take about thirty minutes to cook but are well worth the time and effort. Tinned artichokes hearts are much easier to handle, but they will have lost some of their nutrients.

Jerusalem artichokes are not related to globe artichokes, but are a root vegetable that contain a specific dietary fibre called fructo-oligosaccharides, FOS, which escape digestion and help beneficial lactobacilli ensure that harmful bacteria is removed from the gut. Jerusalem artichokes should be eaten after a course of antibiotics to re-establish the balance of essential bacteria in the gut.

- Asparagus -

In the last few years, cultivation and the shipping of food world-wide has brought the price of asparagus down. Asparagus in common with Jerusalem Artichokes contain FOS. Asparagus contain the antioxidant glutathione. Nearly two thousand years ago, Dioscorides the Greek Physician recommended asparagus as a diuretic.

Asparagus is a natural detoxifier as it increases perspiration and contains sulphur-producing elements that flush the kidneys. The unpleasant sulphurous odour associated with urination after eating asparagus is due to them containing an amino acid called aspartic acid.

A rich source of folate asparagus are an excellent addition to the diet of women in pregnancy.

- Aubergines -

Aubergines, eggplants are purple and glossy, this is due to the antioxidant nasuin found in their skins. An essential part of Indian, Asian and Mediterranean cooking they are a versatile *vegetable* but are best grilled or baked with a little oil; avoid frying them as they are super absorbent and will literally soak up fat. On the plus side they soak up bad cholesterol in the body and are an excellent food containing potassium, vitamin K and vitamin E.

- Beetroot -

The food synonymous with Russia is borscht. I have it on good authority that they make the best borscht in Semipalatinsk, this is the recipe: shred three or four beetroot, chop in their leaves and stalks, cut up an apple and an onion add a potato add two tablespoons of tomato puree. Bring to the boil and simmer for forty minutes.

Beetroot contains, folate, potassium and manganese and the stalk and leaves contain calcium, beta-carotene and iron.

Beetroot are excellent in salads, grated raw or cooked, although they are sweet they have a low calorific value, they are nutrient dense and a vital addition to your diet.

Brussels Sprouts

A member of the cruciferous family they contain cancer fighting antioxidants including indole 3, essential to the working of the intestinal tract. Brussels sprouts contain sulforaphane, which triggers enzymes that help clear the body of toxic waste.

Brussels sprouts strengthen the immune system and the nervous system and help maintain energy levels.

It's essential not to overcook sprouts as with any other vegetables they are best steamed, and eaten al dente.

Part of the traditional Xmas dinner they are far too nutritious to eat on just special occasions. They are an excellent accompaniment to nut roast, roast potatoes, chestnuts and parsnips all the year round.

- Broccoli -

The predominance of broccoli as a popular vegetable is well deserved. It is a superb source of chromium, which helps regulate insulin and blood sugar. High in folate it is another vegetable essential to women in pregnancy. Broccoli is an abundant source of calcium far superior to milk!

Nutritionists have every right to rave about broccoli, as its content of cancer fighting anti-oxidants is truly impressive. It contains indole-3-carbinol, 13C, and sulforaphane that put up a defence against cancer; broccoli is a preventative medicine of the highest order.

Countless laboratory tests have been carried out on broccoli and it is rarely found wanting in any area of disease prevention, it has been found that 13C can lower harmful estrogens that promote tumour growth in hormone sensitive cells, which makes it effective in the fight against breast cancer. Broccoli has also been tested extensively in fighting lung and colon cancer with positive effects.

As with many vegetables it is best eaten raw in salads to get the most of its nutrient value, always choose the darkest green varieties to get the most of its high beta-carotene content which helps convert vitamin A. Raw, steamed or stir-fried it's a food you really should try to eat at least four times a week.

- Crudités -

Crudités are an essential part of your diet, probably the most essential, as there is no limit to how much you eat, or when you decide to snack upon them. If you're looking for the secret of diet success you have found it here. Simply cut up a piece of raw broccoli, a piece of raw cauliflower, a raw carrot, couple of sticks of raw celery, half a raw fennel, a piece of raw cucumber, a few spring onions, and a pepper, and you have the basis of the most invigorating dish on the planet.

Dip them in hummus or virgin olive oil and eat as much as you like in accompaniment with one slice of multi grain wholemeal, or rye bread. You will find that this meal is satisfying and delivers a feeling of wellbeing immediately. You will also find that it difficult to eat this meal in more than human proportions, it's self-regulating!

- Cabbage -

The Romans believed cabbage to be a cure all, they were not far wrong. Like broccoli one of its close relatives it contains, 13C, so it is highly effective in the fight against cancer. Especially in the fight against Colon cancer, as many studies show that even small amounts eaten daily have a beneficial effect. Cabbage contains, iron, calcium and potassium and is a source of Vitamins B1, B2, B3, C and D.

Red cabbage has a higher nutrient value than green and Chinese cabbage contains the compound brassinin, which in laboratory tests has been shown to block cancer.

If you're looking for an interesting way to serve nut roast, when your nut roast is half cooked add some honey and grated ginger to it and wrap, half-portion sizes in cabbage leaves and cook in the oven for twenty minutes.

- Carrots -

Pilots in the RAF in World War II, were served carrots at every opportunity as scientists had discovered that the betacarotene in carrots converts into vitamin A which helps produce the purple pigment called rhodopsin, a light sensitive pigment found in the rod cells of the retina of the eye, essential to night vision.

If that isn't reason enough to eat carrots their vitamin A content also helps fight diseases of the mucous membranes. Research has also shown that betacarotene is highly effective in the fight against heart disease.

Carrots are best eaten raw in salads as when cooked their glycaemic value rises dramatically.

- Celery -

Contains, potassium, calcium and Vitamin C. Celery contains a compound which lowers stress hormones in the blood, which in turn lowers blood pressure. But it should be eaten in moderation, as it contains sodium which eaten to excess raises blood pressure, sometimes getting the balance right is of the utmost importance.

- Cauliflower -

There's a rumour in horticultural circles that broccoli is a hybrid of the cauliflower and the pea. Sometimes the origins of plant life is obscure and can only be traced through DNA.

In the U.K the cauliflower now takes second place to broccoli in its popularity, not the case thirty years ago, when broccoli was more of a seasonal vegetable but the advent of Mediterranean and Chinese cooking brought broccoli to the forefront and it is now imported whenever it cannot be grown locally. Broccoli has placed cauliflower in the shade, which is a shame as its vitamin content make it well worth eating, as does its unique flavour especially raw in crudités.

- Celeriac -

The French adore celeriac, they eat it raw, grated/julienne, as an hors-d'oeuvre. Eaten raw it is full of potassium and soluble fibre that lowers cholesterol, although low in calorific value it is high in sodium which means that it is fine eaten in small amounts.

- Dandelion -

Dandelion is regarded as a weed - it takes root virtually anywhere but it should be treated with more respect, as it is bountiful in Vitamin A, B, C and D. It is also rich in calcium and potassium. The Centurions of Rome prized it highly as do the SAS in their guide to survival. According to Roman physicians, it was a cure-all that covered everything from arthritis to the dissolution of gallstones.

The French treat dandelion with more respect than we do and use it as a salad ingredient.

When removing it from the garden in future, think of it a little differently, a plant only gets the name weed because it grows where it is not wanted. Once you make it a wanted commodity, it ceases to be a weed. Crush and boil the roots to make an infusion that has all the necessary ingredients to lower blood pressure.

87

- Lettuce -

The supermarkets have wasted no time in taking advantage of the generation of people who believe, their time is so valuable that they cannot spare a moment to hold a lettuce under the tap.

Anyone who believes their time is too valuable to hold a lettuce under some cold water needs a reality check.

By pre-packing lettuce the supermarkets have found 'a lovely earner' to quote the sage of Peckham.

Salad should be prepared as close to the time of eating as possible, the cut surfaces of the lettuce loses valuable nutrients, such as folate and vitamin C.

Lettuce leaves should be torn and not cut. Before preparing lettuce it is essential that it is washed thoroughly under cold running water.

Iceberg lettuce, the favourite of fast food chains, as you might expect, is nutritionally far inferior to most other varieties, it retains water and stays in the system twice as long as dark green varieties of salad. Although Iceberg is nutritionally inferior it's economically superior and enhances fast food profits.

Lambs lettuce, baby spinach, rocket and watercress, are the salad ingredients that you need to concentrate on. They should find their way to your table on a regular basis, as they are nutrient rich.

The apothecaries of Rome prized cos/romaine lettuce, as they used the white fluid that seeps from its stalk to calm nerves and promote sleep. Cos/romaine lettuce contains the carotenoid zeaxanthin, to ensure it absorption, it should be eaten with olive oil, in effect the way the Romans ate it. Use olive oil and fresh lemon, as a dressing enhance the nutrients in all dark green salad leaves.

Salads should be as varied as possible and should include, curly endive, chicory, and herbs such as: parsley, sorrel, basil, whatever is available at the time. Add the Asian weed purslane, which has an extremely high level of Omega 3 oils. Add sprouting beans, and you have a salad exploding with nutrients. Sprinkle with sesame, sunflower or pumpkin seeds and add some nuts.

- Garlic -
- Leeks & Onions -

The medicinal properties of garlic have been known for thousands of years. Dried garlic bulbs were found in the tomb of Tutankhamun. When you crush a clove of garlic you release its most potent ingredient allicin, which breaks down fats before they reach the liver.

The Romans used garlic to treat everything from gangrene to respiratory infections. In the 1960's Russia imported tons of garlic to fight a flu epidemic. There have probably been more studies carried out on the beneficial effects of garlic than any other food; its accolades would take a voluminous book to mention.

Studies have show that garlic lowers cholesterol and thins the blood helping to prevent high blood pressure, blocks the growth of cancer cells and has effectively been used in fighting viral infections including encephalitis.

Garlic is used as a medicine world wide, fighting dysentery and typhoid. Whereas we are becoming resistant to synthetic antibiotics, we have not become resistant to the natural antibiotic in garlic.

One of the most alarming thoughts is, as vast areas of rain forest are laid to waste, a plant or root with just a few of the attributes of garlic, not yet discovered, could be destroyed forever.

Garlic is a major part of the Mediterranean diet; recent studies have show that it reduces hardening of the arteries, which to a degree explains Mediterranean longevity.

Garlic's flavour in cooking is unique and it should be used as often as possible, add it wherever you can from soups to salads.

Onions and Leeks contain many of the same properties of garlic but are not as nutritionally dense. As the basis for soups, onions and leeks, bring unique flavours.

Using a non-stick pan, Spanish onions, which are quite sweet, can be fried in the smallest amount of olive oil; onions caramelised this way bring flavour to a dish without losing any nutrients.

Shallots are no afterthought; when you are addicted to their flavour; you find reasons to add them to any dish cooked in the oven.

- Mushrooms -

Cultivated white button mushrooms are an excellent supply of many of the B vitamins, including B12, which is the vitamin that is always cited as lacking in a vegan or a vegetarian diet. They also contain niacin which helps convert sugar into energy.

Anyone who changes from a meat-eating diet to a vegan or vegetarian diet have no immediate need to worry about B12, for quite a while, as the body stores this vitamin for up to three years. Lack of B12 is no problem for a pesco-vegan, as it is amply produced within a balanced diet.

Anyone deciding to take a B12 supplement should ensure that they take B12 in the morning, as when taken late in the day, it can increase energy levels and make it difficult to sleep.

A vast variety of dried fungi are used in oriental medicine, with excellent effects that are now being assiduously studied in the west.

Shitake mushrooms contain the polysaccharide, lentinan, which boosts immunity and builds resistance to bacterial and viral infections.

The Japanese medical establishment use extracts from shitake mushrooms alongside chemotherapy in fighting cancer.

Fresh and dehydrated shitake and maitake mushrooms are now available in your supermarket, they are an excellent addition to soups and vegetarian stews. Try all varieties of oriental mushrooms including enoki and oyster mushrooms. Chestnut mushrooms have an excellent flavour.

Once again healthy diets overlap and the Mediterranean diet utilizes a lot of fresh and dried mushrooms.

Dried mushroom are nutrient dense and should be used sparingly because of their strong taste. Mushrooms should not be eaten raw as they contain toxic chemicals called hydrazines that are eliminated when cooked.

- Parsley -

Parsley contains essential fatty acids, calcium, magnesium and sodium, plus Vitamins A, B and C. Use parsley as much as possible its flavour helps you cut back on salt and its B12 content is important.

After the fad of low-carbohydrate diets is long forgotten we will still be eating and enjoying potatoes.

Baked potatoes in their jackets are reasonably high on the glycaemic index, and should be eaten with low glycaemic foods such as peas or beans, which averages out their glycaemic level, ensuring you get sustained energy as opposed to a burst of energy followed by a low.

Wash and scrub potatoes well before baking them in their jackets, apart from the peel containing some amazing nutrients it also contains an anti-carcinogenic compound called chlorogenic acid which helps the fibre in potatoes bind to any unwanted carcinogens in food.

Potatoes are very high in potassium, which helps maintain blood pressure levels; they also contain vitamins C, B1 and B6.

New Potatoes have a lower glycaemic value and you should have no reservations about making them part of a balanced meal as they have a high satiety level they leave you feeling full.

Sweet potatoes are not a member of the same family of ordinary potatoes, which is the deadly nightshade family. In fact the ordinary potato is closer related to the tomato than the sweet potato, which is part of the morning glory family.

Sweet potatoes contain alpha-carotene and beta-carotene, evolution placed them in just the right place, as they grow in hot climates and reduce skin sensitivity in the people that eat them; they are rich in vitamins C and E.

Sweet potatoes rank highly as they are nutrient dense and amazingly, they are low on the glycaemic index. Mashing ordinary potatoes with sweet potatoes brings down their glycaemic level and increases the nutrient level of your meal.

Chop in as much fresh parsley as you can when mashing these potatoes together with a little olive oil, as beta-carotene needs fat to get it through the intestinal wall. These ingredients placed together constitute the true meaning of a balanced meal.

" What I say is that if a man really likes potatoes,
he must be a pretty decent sort of a fellow"
- A A Milne.

- Radish -

The sheer fact that radish is a relative of broccoli should be enough of a nutritional endorsement. Popular amongst ancient cultures from the Chinese to the Egyptians they are exceptional as a diuretic and are used extensively in herbal medicine. Radishes are simple to grow, even in a window box, and their leaves can be boiled and used as an infusion to fight respiratory infections.

- Radicchio -

Radicchio, Italian for red chicory, is rich in vitamins B and C and is rich in iron, phosphorous and calcium. As part of a salad radicchio enhances the dark green leaves of lambs lettuce, watercress and baby spinach, in both appearance and nutrients. Eat radicchio the way the Venetians do by steaming it for the shortest time and serve it with rice, use brown basmati rice and ensure that you add some olive oil at the last moment to enhance the nutrients.

- Rice -

Rice is one of the planets staple foods of which there are over 40,000 varieties worldwide. Try as many varieties of brown rice as you can, eventually you will discover the rice that suits you best. Brown rice is fibre rich and will keep cholesterol levels down.

Polished rice, white rice, is nutritionally inferior to brown rice, as it doesn't contain the levels of oryzanol, the compound that lowers cholesterol. Numerous studies have shown that colon cancer is virtually unknown in populations whose staple diet is brown rice.

Cooking rice is an art, cook it gently and let it absorb as much water as possible, also add fresh herbs late in the cooking process as the rice will absorb their nutrients. The more you experiment with cooking the more adventurous you are going to get, your only restriction in creating new dishes is your imagination!

- Peppers & Chillies -

The traffic light colours of bell peppers, red, yellow and green enhance salads and stir-fries. Left whole and stuffed with lentils and butter beans, rice and peas or nut roast, they illustrate how interesting vegan or vegetarian food can be.

Peppers are nutrient dense with vitamin C and beta-carotene. To ensure maximum nutritional value and that the betacarotene is absorbed add olive oil. Eat peppers often, as with all nutrient dense foods they must go to the top of your list. Peppers contain the natural pain killer capsaicin, and are a favoured food of endurance athletes, who need all the help they can get in passing the pain barrier.

Chillies are excellent for flavouring, add them to rice and you can devise dishes that could have originated in Eastern Europe or Asia, cooking interesting food is about three things, nutritious ingredients, improvisation and timing.

- Spinach -

Spinach is essential for salads and as a cooked vegetable it takes less than a minute to steam. Its nutrients are astounding, as with all leafy green vegetables, we need to eat them daily. They are at the basis of our wellbeing, everything that green vegetables are, junk food isn't!

Don't miss out on any dark green vegetable. Brussels tops, young spring greens, sprouting broccoli, and of course spinach. They contain an abundance of: magnesium, iron, calcium, folate, lutein, betacarotene and vitamins C and B6.

To be at the top of our physical form, we need to ensure that we eat these vegetables at every opportunity.

I apologise for repeating myself, but I have had to physically restrain myself from not making a third reiteration of this very important mantra.

Snow Peas & Mange Tout

An essential in stir-fries they take seconds to cook, and an excellent addition to salads; they are fibre rich.

- Marrows & Courgettes -

The marrow and the courgette cannot boast much in the way of nutrients, although they contain betacarotene, vitamin C and folate.

We have very little interest in calorific values, but purely academically, they don't contain many calories. Marrows make an excellent dish stuffed with rice or lentils and finely sliced courgettes are wonderful in stir-fries, their skins are highly nutritious.

- Pumpkin -

Considering the nutritional density in pumpkin seeds, already covered earlier, it will come as no surprise that pumpkins are one of the most nutritious foods on the planet.

A main part of the Thanksgiving Day meal, pumpkins need to be incorporated into your diet as often as possible. Pumpkins brim with cancer fighting antioxidants. They contain some of the more elusive carotenoids, such as lutein and zeaxanthin, essential to healthy eyesight and blocking the formation of cataracts. The properties in pumpkins fight a whole range of cancers. Not surprisingly with such a powerful nutrient content their taste is strong, to ameliorate their taste, use fresh orange or fresh lime-juice.

- Fennel -

Hippocrates advised nursing mothers to eat fennel. On the Island of Crete his advice is still heeded. The Cretans, before the advent of junk food held the record for longevity of all Mediterranean countries.

Menopausal women benefit from the diuretic properties in fennel, as it is also rich in phytoestrogens and folate.

When selecting fennel go for the female variety as they have much more flavour, they are easily determined as they are more rounded at the base. Fennel is an exceptional food; cooked for a few moments under the grill, with a little olive oil, it is a wonderful accompaniment to grilled fish. Eaten raw dipped in olive oil, along with green yellow and red peppers it is invigorating; you should be able to feel its beneficial effects - as you eat it!

- Ginger -
& The Chinese Connection

The Chinese regard ginger as a highly potent medicine and have done for thousands of years. When the Roman Legions travelled by ship, they took ginger to alleviate motion sickness. If you suffer from motion sickness, try it – it usually works!

Chinese medical practitioners recommend it for everything from upset stomach, to migraines. Ginger is an excellent anti-inflammatory, anti-depressant and anti-coagulant. Open a Chinese doctors' bag and don't be surprised if all you find - is a piece of ginger.

A hot drink made with ginger and manuka honey will soothe you through viral infections. Use ginger in your cooking, apart from adding that taste of the orient it will stimulate your metabolism.

The best place to buy ginger is your local Chinese store, as they will not have any substandard ginger for sale, their customers are far too astute to entertain anything but the best.

Look a little deeper at everything when you get to your Chinese store, simple things like sets of bamboo steamers are excellent for sprouting seeds.

Rich sauces loaded with additives are to be avoided, but look closely at their vegetables. This is an excellent place to buy varieties of dried mushrooms, Chinese turnips, water chestnuts and exotic varieties of beans tinned and dried. If you are going to buy a wok this is the place. Food knows no frontiers! This is the place to expand your horizons, don't be afraid to ask how something is cooked, you're dealing with an ancient culture that loves to impart information.

- Green Tea -

Green tea is flavour of the month the year and the decade. The only thing better than green tea is white tea, which is ten times the price as it can only be picked for a few days in the year.

Green tea is a powerful anti-oxidant. If you're interested in longevity, you've found your drink. When in your local Chinese store, buy the gunpowder variety. Get used to green tea, as you should be drinking it well into your nineties. Keep a teapot full by your side!

- Chocolate -

Chocolate is not a no go area, as long as it is chocolate you are buying and not some adulterated, well advertised, substance that is full of hydrogenated fat and sugar.

It has to be dark and at least, seventy percent cocoa. Chocolate as with all nutrient rich foods needs to be eaten in moderation, instead of attempting to overdo it, eat a quarter of a bar with fresh fruit, dried fruit and nuts. This way you are going to get the most from a nutrient dense treat and you don't have to have a psychological battle with yourself, dating back to when you had some awful misapprehension about food.

Chocolate contains folic acid, copper, potassium, magnesium and B vitamins. Studies published in The Lancet have shown that chocolate contains polyphenols, which protect against heart disease.

Chocolate also contains phenylethylamine and theobromine that boost serotonin levels. It affects the same areas of the brain as sex.

Anyone trying to give up chocolate is fighting a losing and unnecessary battle, eating chocolate in moderation is fine; it's a sensuous experience. It melts in your mouth and evokes the most pleasurable eating experiences of childhood.

Buy 'Fairtrade' chocolate wherever possible, Green & Blacks sell an organic variety that ensures farmers and growers are not exploited.

- Carob -

Carob has a lot less fat content to chocolate and is a lot less satisfying. In its favour it doesn't have the caffeine content of chocolate and it is protein rich. It is high in calcium and is rich in vitamins A and B. When making chocolate cakes, a mixture of chocolate and carob enhances the nutrient value, ensure you use wholemeal flour!

" Page one is a diet, page two is a chocolate cake,
It's a no win situation!"
- Kim Williams   writing about 'women's magazines.'

Herbs & Spices

The microwave and corkscrew contingent do not have much use for herbs and spices and it would take a volume and somebody really versed in the art to do herbs and spices justice.

These days you can buy fresh herbs growing in pots, in your supermarket, at least they have managed to get something right.

The way the best chefs approach their cooking is by seeing what is available and building their menu around the fresh produce that is reasonable and plentiful. They don't march off with a shopping list; they improvise and gain inspiration. If you're in the supermarket and a pot of basil catches your eye, start thinking of basil and tomato soup.

Spontaneity is what makes great dishes. When adding herbs to your food, always add them as late as possible, mixed dried herbs enhance roasted vegetables. Fresh rosemary and roasted parsnips, a vegetable I neglected to list (highly glycaemic but full of potassium) is the centrepiece of a table field with roasted vegetables and nut roast.

In the west we know little of the value of spices, but there is nothing to stop us learning; a wonderful instance is cinnamon.

- Cinnamon -

The journal of Diabetes Care found that a half-teaspoon of cinnamon taken daily significantly reduces blood sugar levels in people with type two diabetes. It also reduced triglycerides, LDL cholesterol and total cholesterol levels amongst diabetics.

Cinnamon is an anti-inflammatory and an anticoagulant it helps stimulate circulation and relieves menstrual pains. It is also a powerful anti-microbial that kills E Coli and other bacteria. Stir a cinnamon stick into your green tea and it will raise your metabolism.

- Cloves -

Oil of cloves, rubbed directly onto the gums, relieves toothache Just taking this instance as a guide of how powerful one spice can be in relieving substantial pain, what might you be missing with many others? Spices have to be added to your cooking repertoire.

The Latter and the Former

Transition is different for each individual, many will make the necessary changes to prevent becoming ill, many will wait for some kind of physical warning, that all is not well, I hope you are the former.

The human brain is an amazing creation, we run around looking to upgrade our computer to the latest model, when we have the finest possible upgrade sitting neglected under our hat. To have been gifted something as remarkable as the human brain, and to then feed it on garbage is sacrilege. Feeding the brain with nutrients is more important than reading the right books, as the latter can only be achieved by pursuing the former.

Allowing children to eat junk food is a chronic waste of amazing potential, sending a child to school without an adequate breakfast, means they will not be able to function at an optimum level, they will be tired and lethargic and their school work will suffer. This is not fantasy - this is scientifically proven fact.

Overall, real-food is far cheaper than non-food, so there is no economic excuse. It takes a little more effort, but there can be no greater example to a child than a parent who makes a sustained effort.

If in the past you did not realise that a bowl of cornflakes and milk was non-food, you are blameless, but once the 'Truth About Food' is implicit, placing the onus on children to make informed decisions about food is unfair, as they can only see as far as the cornflake packet on the table and for many of them, it is the only thing they are given to read. From an early age that list of ingredients on the cornflakes packet is what they perceive to be food.

A child's nourishment and wellbeing is the responsibility of the parent, and we in the western world are so fortunate that ample sustenance is available. Children can only be educated by example!

" If your are planning for a year, sow rice,
if you are planning for a decade, plant trees,
if you are planning for a lifetime, educate people."
- Chinese Proverb

The Price of Rice

There isn't a recipe in the world that cannot be modified to use real-food, it takes some ingenuity but it is well worth the effort.

Replacing saturated and trans fats with, walnut or almond oil makes it possible to bake wonderful cakes, providing you replace white flour with wholemeal flour. Using coconut butter, coconut milk, soya milk, rice milk or oat milk - and honey to sweeten, means that there's not much you can't achieve, with a little imagination and a cornucopia of dried fruit, nuts and spices.

People talk of the Mediterranean diet as if it is some abstract concept that just occurs. It transpires because the whole family becomes involved in the kitchen. In a French, Greek, Italian or Spanish kitchen, every member of the family has an informed opinion of how food should be prepared. It's a life enhancing event, not the opening of some sterile packet from the supermarket, with a studio photograph of a meal on its outside, that is then *cooked* in a microwave oven.

You have to reclaim what is rightfully yours, the right to real-food, good wholesome food that you prepare yourself, not something manufactured in a soulless factory.

Go to your local greengrocer, buy your produce fresh and cook it on the same day, visit your local fishmonger and whenever possible buy 'fair-trade' produce. Instigate change for the better!

Once upon a time we could tell when prices were marked-up by the price sticker on our purchase; but with the advent of bar codes, prices rise electronically overnight. If you stopped a hundred people in the street and asked them the price of a loaf of bread most of them would look at you in amazement.

How have we allowed ourselves to become so sophisticated that we do not know the price of a loaf of bread?

It is time to become the person who decides exactly what they buy as opposed to the gullible consumer, willing to have non-food surreptitiously foisted upon them.

> " *The superior man knows what is right,*
> *the inferior man knows what sells.* "
> - Confucius

The Same Old Story

On the day prior to this book going to press 19th March 2004, Coca Cola recalled its new, bottled *'pure water,'* ordinary tap water with a mark-up of an unbelievable 300,000 percent. Coca Cola's *enhanced-purification* process contaminated pure tap water with cancer causing bromate. This monumental mistake, superseded by the mother of all mark-ups, is just about the saddest reflection of the non-food industry, which treats its customers with unbelievable contempt.

The non-food industry and the diet industry feed off each other, and are equally contemptuous of the consumer; they believe it is their right to perpetuate the lucrative situation they find themselves in.

At this very moment someone somewhere is trying to think up a new gimmick, that they can expand into a wonder diet, knowing there are many desperate people out there who will try anything to lose weight. But every *new* angle they come up with, only involves the same old story, adding and subtracting various foods and backing up the notion with a barrage of pseudo-psychology and false hope.

There is no need for anyone to be a victim of a system that has been allowed to spiral out of control. Return to basics, return to simplicity, eat real-food in human proportions, eat nutrient rich food four times a day, exercise daily and you will become fitter and stronger in mind and body. Completely reclaim your own existence!

Enthuse about real-food to your friends and family; help them to understand 'The Truth About Food.' This is a proven diet that people have thrived on for thousands of years. Good health and longevity are the right of every person on this planet!

" Tell me and I'll forget, show me, I may remember,
involve me and I'll understand"
- Chinese Proverb.